Nursing Care:
the challenge
to change

NURSING CARE:
the challenge
to change

Edited by

Moya Jolley
**MA(Ed), BSc(Econ), SRN, Dip Ed, RNT, Dip in Nursing
(Lond)**
Lecturer, Sociology and Nursing Development,
Institute of Advanced Nursing Education, Royal College
of Nursing, London

and

Gosia Brykczyńska
BSc, BA, RGN, RSCN, Dip PH, Cert Ed, ONC Cert
Lecturer, Nursing Studies, Institute of Advanced
Nursing Education, Royal College of Nursing, London

Edward Arnold
A division of Hodder & Stoughton
LONDON MELBOURNE AUCKLAND

© 1992 the contributors listed on page xi

First published in Great Britain 1992

British Library Cataloguing in Publication Data
A CIP catalogue record for this title
is available from the British Library

ISBN 0 340 53920 8

Typeset in Linotron Times by
Rowland Phototypesetting Limited, Bury St Edmunds, Suffolk
Printed and bound in Great Britain for Edward Arnold, a division
of Hodder and Stoughton Limited, Mill Road, Dunton Green,
Sevenoaks, Kent TN13 2YA by
Biddles Limited, Guildford and King's Lynn

Foreword

'The distinction between being a moral philosopher and being a nurse is primarily that a nurse must act upon her moral conclusions, the philosopher need not.' With these words, Eileen Inglesby sums up the significance of this book. For they highlight the challenge which confronts every practising nurse. Every day, every hour, nurses are involved in decisions and practices which are based on ethical criteria and which have far-reaching ethical implications. And as new knowledge and skills increase the opportunities to save life and to prevent death, nurses will become increasingly involved in moral choices which will have profound effects on their patients and clients, their families and the community.

These opportunities and the challenges which accompany them mean that these are exciting days for nursing. As nursing develops professionally, with more autonomy and independence, the moral responsibility for decisions and actions also increases. It is therefore imperative that nurses are equipped to understand essential moral issues and to think critically about the ethical assumptions underlying their own professional practice.

New educational initiatives in the development of Project 2000 courses will enable students to have the time and the opportunity to study ethical issues and to think critically about the assumptions and implications of that elusive concept of 'care' which lies at the heart of nursing. Much has been written already, but much has not been directly relevant or useful for British students: e.g. American work does not always easily transpose into British situations; and much of the thinking to date has not proved adequate for direct transfer to practice. Some theories are so abstract or so partial that they are unsuitable for direct application, and have sometimes been embraced with over-enthusiastic naivete in ways which will do little to help the quality of patient care. For example, I will never forget visiting a hospital in another country where the nursing leaders had whipped up a frenzy of activity in organising a ballot amongst all nursing staff to determine by vote whether the nursing throughout the hospital should be based on the theories of Orem or of Roy. This simplistic and totally inappropriate use of nursing 'theories' illustrates the urgent need for nurses as a profession to understand the essential philosophical and ethical underpinnings of practice.

This book offers a splendid basis for critical thinking about the ethical implications of the care which constitutes nursing practice. Its readable summaries of key works; its balanced and thoughtful accounts of key issues and its use of real-life examples, with their human poignancy, should make the study of the ethical implications of care rewarding and stimulating for the present generation of students whose responsibilities will require them to be accountable according to criteria which include complex moral as well as legal dimensions.

The first chapter discusses five elements of the concept of 'care' itself: compassion, competence, conscience, commitment and confidence. Gosia Brykczynska weaves together themes from standard nursing texts with those from classical literature to illustrate the timelessness and universality of aspects of the human predicament; she reminds the reader that no amount of theory will compensate for incompetence in practical clinical skills, although these need to be understood in a wider frame of knowledge; she also discusses the importance of confidence – the nurse's own professional confidence (which must be well-founded and not confused with inappropriate assertiveness) and the patient's confidence in the nurse, based on a relationship of trust engendered by the nurses's personal commitment. The chapter reflects the myriad challenges and satisfactions which make nursing unique.

Other chapters provide useful overviews of key topics which are relevant to ethical aspects of nursing: a discussion of the values which underpin nursing; the importance of quality assurance in determining the extent to which nursing practice is both care-effective and cost-effective; the contribution of information systems and information technology to high standards and efficient management of resources.

The final chapter discusses a subject often neglected in today's increasingly secular Western society: the spiritual dimension of nursing care. If nursing claims to provide 'holistic' care, we are reminded that we cannot ignore 'the wounded soul'. Whatever each individual nurses's own beliefs may be, there is a moral imperative to attend to a patient's spiritual needs and not to evade or avoid those concerns which may be causing great distress. The commitment to companionship with another person undergoing the agony of spiritual distress can be an ultimate challenge, but one which is an integral part of care. There may be no removal of problems, no answers to questions, or no solution to suffering, but the nurse can comfort by compassionate atttentiveness. This chapter also deals sensitively with issues such as therapeutic touch, respect for the healing potential of beauty, the importance of learning to care for each other, and the value of humour.

I cannot help feeling a little envious of the students who, while they are preparing to become qualified nurses, will have the opportunity to read this book and to benefit from its rich source of ideas and wisdom! My envy however, is tempered by respect for them and for the awesome responsibilities they will face as they move into a world of nursing which is going to require them to think ever more critically about the care they give and which will challenge them in ever more demanding ways. For them, this book will be not only stimulating, but immensely valuable.

Baroness Cox of Queensbury
Deputy Speaker
House of Lords

Contents

List of contributors

Gosia Brykczyńska BSc, BA, RGN, RSCN, Dip.PH, Cert Ed, ONC Cert
Lecturer, Nursing Studies, Institute of Advanced Nursing Education, Royal College of Nursing, London

Eileen Inglesby BA(Hons), Cert Ed, SRN, RNT
Freelance Lecturer and Writer

Betty Kershaw MSc, SRN, RCNT, RNT, DANS, OND
Principal, Stockport, Thameside and Glossop College of Nursing, Stockport

Kim Manley MN, RGN, Dip in Nursing, RCNT
Lecturer, Nursing Studies, Institute of Advanced Nursing Education, Royal College of Nursing, London

Diane Marks-Maran BSc, SRN, Dip in Nursing (Lond), RNT
Director of Curriculum, Queen Charlotte's College of Health Care Studies, Ealing Hospital, Middlesex

Rosalind Rundle MA, BA, RGN, RHV, SCM, FWT Cert, PGCEA
Lecturer, Health Studies, Institute of Advanced Nursing Education, Royal College of Nursing, London

Angela Trueman JP, MA, BA, RGN, ONC, Dip in Nursing (Lond), Cert Ed, RNT
Vice Principal, Dept of Education and Training, Royal Marsden Hospital, London

Preface

At the present time an ever increasing number of students are under-taking advanced courses in nursing. This developing trend suggests that there is a need for a shift in textbook literature away from the more generalised preparatory texts to those providing a degree of in-depth analysis of pertinent nursing issues. British nurses, studying nursing art and science, find themselves engaged in the process of endeavouring to familiarise themselves with both nursing research, and nursing theory. The awkward problem frequently arises of then having to choose from a selection of either very basic introductory texts, sometimes providing somewhat simplified approaches to nursing theory and research, or texts that require the student to make a considerable intellectual leap forward, for which they may not yet be adequately prepared. Such texts include works on nursing theory, written for the most part by senior American nurse theorists for an American academic readership. These monographs may be seen by some nurses as too far removed from the British reality of nursing to be of any great practical assistance.

This book seeks to address the problem stated above by providing a middle range text having relevance for students taking Project 2000 courses, as well as those taking degree and diploma courses in nursing studies.

A range of nursing issues are addressed, many of which constitute the core of modern British nursing thought. All chapters are both independent from, yet interrelated to each other, and are written by experts in their respective subject fields. Nursing theory, nursing process, ethics, information systems and quality assurance are each addressed and critically evaluated within the overall framework of caring as an art in the modern British context.

It is the hope of the editors that this book will be of assistance to all students of nursing seeking to enhance their knowledge and skills in professional practice.

London
January 1992

Moya Jolley
Gosia Brykczyńska

Acknowledgements

The editors would like to extend their grateful thanks to all the contributors to this book. Their expertise, generosity in time and energy, as well as enthusiasm and commitment, have made this book possible.

Thanks go also to Baroness Cox for writing the Foreword; and to Miss Maria Bnińska in assisting in manuscript preparation.

Appreciation and thanks are also extended to Miss Helen Thomas, Assistant Librarian in the Library of Nursing at the RCN, for her meticulous work in checking and preparing references, and her unflagging professional support. Also to Mrs Jean Smith for her tireless efforts, great patience and unfailing support in the preparation of the final manuscript. Last but not least, we would like to thank Nancy Loffler for her continued support and generous help with this publication.

1 Caring – a dying art?

Caring as a concept is elusive. Although all humans need caring in order to mature into healthy well-functioning adults, the nurturing aspects of caring behaviours are neither self-evident nor inevitable. Gaylin (1976) and the social anthropologists often highlight the naturalness of nurturing behaviours, but caring as a concept used by professional carers, especially nurses, is far wider in its meaning and far more complex to analyse.

Morse (1990) in a brilliant review of caring theories, as postulated and used by nurses, aptly points out that in order to make sense of the ever-growing literature on caring, it is necessary to be able to classify and codify the concepts and constructs of caring. In that respect and caring-analysts will have a chance to identify their relevant perspectives, and critics of the 'caring theories' can be somewhat appeased that efforts are being made to define terms, delineate boundaries of concern and identify areas of semantic and ideological difficulties (Morse *et al*; 1990; Smith, 1990; Dunlop, 1986; Boykin and Schoenhofer, 1980; Watson, 1988).

Morse identifies at least five major caring perspectives, in which caring theories often overlap and sustain credence by being seen in apposition to one or more of the other theories of the main caring perspectives.

Caring is being discussed by many professionals (Gaylin, 1976; Campbell, 1984; Mayeroff, 1971), and some nursing professionals like Delores Gaut (1983) have been striving for over a decade to describe adequately the nature of professional caring. As Gaut (1983) notes:

> 'A theoretically adequate description of any concept requires not only clarification of the constituents of the concept that can generate or derive any instance of the concept, but also must speak of the relationship between the constituents.'

It is the intention of this chapter and the subsequent chapters in this book, to elucidate nursing care, to make more clear what is understood by caring behaviour, how efficient and expert nursing practice can promote caring, and how all the various constituents of nursing care have a role to play in nurses' caring acts.

Firstly, it needs to be emphasised that not all nurse theorists perceive a need to analyse caring as thoroughly as Gaut (1981, 1983, 1984, 1986).

Leininger (1986) states unequivocally that:

1

'Nursing is caring; caring is the heart of nursing; and care can be a powerful means of healing and promoting healthy life ways.'

(Leininger, 1986; p. 3)

She considers care to be the central and distinct phenomenon of nursing. Gaut, however, uses an action description of caring. She is concerned with methods of evaluating competencies required in caring actions and she considers caring to be an intentional human enterprise (Gaut, 1986). She explains that her

'competency model of caring goes beyond the identification of just observable performative skills to include broader considerations such as intention, choices and judgments that underlie the performance.'

(Gaut, 1986; p. 82)

Watson in her works on caring identifies seven basic assumptions in the science of caring in nursing, the first of which is that caring can be effectively demonstrated and practised only interpersonally. Like Leininger she sees the practice of caring as central to nursing, and in attempting to define caring professionalism in nursing practice lists ten primary caring factors such as the need for a humanistic-altruistic system of values, the instillation of faith-hope, and the systematic use of scientific problem-solving methods for decision-making, among others.

Ray (1981) in her paper on *A philosophical analysis of caring within nursing* writes of caring as a 'form of loving oblative or other directed love, where co-presence in human encounter is a mystery rather than a problem to be solved' (Ray, 1981, p. 32).

Finally, Roach, who sees that her 'reflections on caring have evolved primarily from a philosophical and theological perspective', describes caring in the first instance as 'an essential human attribute' (Roach, 1985; p. 170). She sees caring 'operationalised in nursing through the specific attributes of compassion, competence, confidence, conscience and commitment' (Roach, 1985; p. 171). For Roach, 'caring is living in the context of relational responsibilities' (Roach, 1985; p. 176) which is why she echoes Mayeroff's observation that 'caring, as helping another grow and actualise himself, is a process, a way of relating to someone that involves *development*, in the same way that friendship can only emerge through mutual trust and a deepening and qualitative transformation of the relationship' (Mayeroff, 1971; p. 1). Interestingly Parse (1981) defines caring in a similar vein as 'risking being with someone towards a moment of joy', and Campbell (1985), defining pastoral care as a kind of loving, states that care has one fundamental aim: 'to help people to know love, both as something to be received and as something to give' (Campbell, 1985; p. 1).

Nurse theorists and educationalists, even if they have difficulty in defining care, are adamant however, about its intrinsic value and place within the profession of nursing. Thus Cooper (1990) considers that nurses see care as the 'ethical standard by which even *cure* is measured' (emphasis mine), and Darbyshire (1990) would like to have care introduced into nursing models of practice and curricula, since he fears that:

> 'the frequently heard complaint of "burn-out" is a good example of what can happen when we lose our ability to care, when things and people no longer matter and become the mere objects of our supposedly professional attentions.'
>
> (Darbyshire, 1990)

As he points out, in communion with the majority of 'caring-theory' advocates, 'Caring about someone or something elevates the carer to the position where previously unseen aspects become relevant, meaningful and important' (Darbyshire, 1990). Griffin in her paper on *Philosophical Analysis of Caring in Nursing* additionally notes that 'in caring for a patient, unlooked for benefits may accrue to a nurse' for it is a great privilege, as she rightly contends 'to be with a human being at his most vulnerable, where appearances and descriptions no longer mask personality, and where everything most valuable – life or whatever makes it most meaningful – is being risked' (Griffin, 1983).

Others like Fry (1988) and Moccia (1988) point out the potential courage and social activism that caring adequately for another may engender. Moccia observes that 'given the crises we face, nursing's intertwining tradition of caring and radical change is needed now more than ever' (Moccia, 1988). That it may take courage to care genuinely for someone may be understandable, but as a consequence of our recent emphasis on individualised nursing care and greater involvement with patients, it is now becoming more evident that there is an emotional cost to pay also (Smith, 1991; Hutchinson, 1990; Pepper, 1985).

Certainly caring is considered on the one hand 'a natural state of being' and on the other a skilled learned art that demands much forethought, education, and moral integrity. No wonder theorists like Smith (1990) ask how it can be that caring is both ubiquitous and unique – as she puts it:

> 'If the stance is taken that caring is a core concept unique to nursing, then why do so many claim it? . . . how can a universal experience be at the core of a particular science when it is difficult to specify the meaning of it?
>
> (Smith, 1990)

Dunlop in 1986 queried whether a science of caring is possible, given the difficulties in defining and describing professional caring. Dunlop rightly states that it is the depersonalisation of the health-care system that has led to the emergence of caring as a construct within nursing, the 'enriched meaning of caring which is emerging can be seen as a way of attempting to solve the problem' (Dunlop, 1986). Finally she cautions would-be caring enthusiasts to be mindful of their concepts and conceptual parameters; 'while it seems possible to claim that nursing is a form of caring, it seems much less reasonable to claim it as *the* form of caring' (Dunlop, 1986).

It is the caring aspects of nursing, however, which can be taught, that interest educationalists (Forsyth *et. al*; 1989; Leininger and Watson, 1990). From ethicists like Carper (1979) to theorists such as Watson (1988) and Gaut (1986) nursing professionalism is being redefined along moral and yet simultaneously functional-analytical lines. Caring is being given an ever greater role to play in the determinants of clinical excellence and expertise. Whether Boykin and Schoenhofer's (1990) five categories of caring theories are used or Morse's (1990), it is abundantly clear that in order to analyse nursing practice in the 1990s, there will be a need for an understanding of caring theories and how caring as human purposeful activity shapes the moral integrity of nursing interventions. Liehr (1989) opens her short paper on *True Presence – a Loving Center* with the statement:

> 'As one matures in nursing, it becomes increasingly clear that the unique gift a nurse has to offer is to share self by being truly present with another.'
>
> (Liehr, 1989)

This unique gift of self shared with another has been called by others, true caring, and to sustain this gift of self there is the need for professional devotion. Mayeroff notes that when 'devotion breaks down caring breaks down' (Mayeroff, 1971; p. 8).

Roach (1985) by closely examining the concept of caring has formulated a foundation for moral nursing practice based on five elements of caring behaviour; compassion, competence, confidence, conscience and commitment. The remainder of this chapter will examine her five elements of caring behaviours and in so doing demonstrate why sometimes caring breaks down, and how caring aspects of nurses' work can be improved. As Roach notes:

> 'the nurse does not "deliberate" about whether or not she ought to care, for to care is the end of nursing. She deliberates on how caring can best be accomplished.'
>
> (Roach, 1985)

Caring can best be accomplished by a concerted effort at integration of appropriate philosophies, and research findings; nursing's evaluative processes such as quality assurance schemes; application of systematic approaches to nursing such as the nursing process within models of nursing; and a keenness to utilise new techniques and labour saving equipment such as computers and information technology, whether in the community or in a hospital context. All these professional nursing issues will be addressed in this book. It is the intention of this chapter, however, to demonstrate, as Alison Kitson wrote earlier:

> 'A consciousness of caring would seem to grow from within the person and also from without. We cannot care without having been cared for, nor can we care without first having sensed what matters to us, what makes us want to care. Whatever matters to us structures our world and determines our interest in things and relations with others.'
>
> (Kitson, 1985)

Compassion

Professional compassion is a form of 'moderated love', a very powerful feeling which is of fundamental importance to the practitioner of nursing. It tends to propel the practitioner into a caring mode (Campbell, 1984). As Gaylin notes in his essay on *Feelings*, 'feelings are the fine instruments that shape decision-making in an animal cursed and blessed with intelligence and the freedom which is its corollary . . . ' (Gaylin, 1985). Feeling compassionate towards a stranger followed up by an empathetic approach is a necessary pre-requisite for true caring to take place and, given that the presence of the feeling is its own reward; a positive feedback mechanism is set into motion. Gaylin assures us that 'feelings are internal directives essential for human life. In addition and not just in passing, they are their own rewards. They are the means and the ends' (Gaylin, 1985).

Of all the constructs of caring, perhaps the one that most readily comes to mind is compassion. We feel that at a minimum, to care at some yet to be determined level, must involve compassion.

Compassion is seen to encompass more than just the notions of pity or concern; and certainly dictionary definitions imply that compassion is a shared attribute of caring, for to show or have compassion involves suffering with another. Whether or not it is possible to ever share 'another's sorrow' is a moot point, a philosophical question discussed at length by moral philosophers from Plato to Iris Murdoch (Hamilton and Cairns, 1961; Murdoch, 1970). Hare, in his critique of Murdoch's anti-utilitarian position, in deliberating on the nature and extent of empathy that is necessary if compassion is to be exercised, makes much effort to delineate the difference between 'knowing that something is happening to someone, and knowing what it is like for him' (Hare, 1981). Often in nursing a particular patient we have a fairly good idea of what is physiologically occurring with the patient, but very rarely can we actually know what it is *like for them*. The nurse who has never herself breast-fed her baby may know on a cognitive level physiologically and even psychologically what may be occurring to the young mother who is attempting to put her first-born child to the breast – but the act itself will always remain difficult for the non-parous woman to identify with. Here the affective and cognitive states are discordant and there certainly is room for an argument that maintains that at some level no-one can ever really *know* what even common life experiences can be like for another person. One person's lived experience, per definition, is unique, and empathy in such a context must limit itself at best to a partial understanding. When the empathy concerns a situation that falls within the general domain of collective life experiences, such as loss of a spouse, often sufficient numbers of people have had a similar experience. The experience now does not appear exceptional, and can be at least superficially incorporated into the world-view of the other. Interestingly, nurses are often heard to say, 'I thought I knew what it was like, until I lost my own husband; now I *really* know'.

The nurse in such an example is stating the central paradox of empathy – that in order to really adequately empathise, one needs to go through a similar experience oneself. However, even a similar experience will never be the *same* experience, for it is not the life event as such that one is identifying with. That can be done reasonably adequately on a purely cognitive level. What is required in empathy is a sufficient projection of self into the private world of the other, to be able (at least partially) to understand *effectively* what the experience means for *them*. This, however, is not the same thing as considering how *I* would feel in a given situation. Such an undertaking would be a useful exercise in a clarification of values, but would yield only limited information about ourselves, and how we might behave in a similar circumstance.

This distinction is brought out very well by Hare who took the example of suffering as an ego state worthy of examination (Hare, 1981). He states it is imperative to appreciate the distinction in the experience of suffering between affective and cognitive states 'in particular between suffering, and knowing that I am suffering' (Hare, 1981; p. 92). Hare claims that in the state of suffering the cognitive and affective mode come together, although he sees the possibility for some individuals affectively to know suffering, but not to do so cognitively. 'It has to be admitted that a being, if there were such, who lacked self-consciousness might suffer without knowing that it was *he* who suffered' (Hare, 1981).

Such a situation is not uncommon with a seriously ill unconscious patient, or a young severely multiply-handicapped child. In such a situation personal suffering is experienced globally and diffusely, and there is little or minimal psychic or spiritual involvement in the suffering. An otherwise healthy infant can also experience global suffering, but this is a total body and soul distress, such as when its heel is lanced in order to obtain a drop of blood for analysis. This suffering is, however, simultaneously limitless and all encompassing for the infant. The experience is completely beyond the truly empathetic reach of an adult.

Hare also points out that 'suffering' as a term is often used interchangeably with concepts of pain. Meanwhile the literature suggests that suffering as a manifestation of total distress includes concepts of pain, but itself has much wider connotations. Suffering, according to Hare, brings together the affective and cognitive states, but also the conative state, and it is this desire and drive to end the suffering, (to see it as something negative), that is projected sufficiently strongly by the sufferer and is interpreted by the nurse. The empathetic nurse can then recognise the 'suffering state', and therefore become compassionate in her caring for the patient.

Gaylin points out that emotions are contagious, and a display of emotions such as empathy and compassion serves the purpose of making the concerned carer aware that help is needed,

'. . . even without knowing why, we respond to the feelings of others. Emotions are contagious . . . they are not just directives to ourselves but directives from others to us, indicating that we have been seen, that we have been understood, that we have been appreciated, that we have made contact.'

(Gaylin, 1985)

In order to empathise one must, as Hare explains, consider what it is like to be somebody else who is suffering. In order to empathise truly, the knowing and understanding of another must include knowledge and understanding of *their* preferences in *that* situation:

'I need to imagine myself in his situation with his preferences. Unless I have an equal aversion to myself suffering, forthwith, what he is suffering or going to suffer, I cannot really be knowing, or even believing, that being in his situation with his preferences will be like *that*.'

(Hare, 1981; p. 95)

The nurse in part of her compassionate care is called to be empathetic, but what is less often discussed is how the professionally disinterested nurse is to find the inner resources to be at least even partially empathetic (Barber, 1991). Hare did not suggest that true empathy is possible; in fact he alluded to such possibilities occurring only among archangels. He suggested mortals may find true empathy difficult in practice, but an attempt at even partial acquisition of such skills is useful, if not desirable, should we wish to act morally and to help in the analysing of morally distressing situations. Thus:

> 'It is the latter kind of knowledge (of empathy) which, I am proposing, we should treat as relevant, and as required for the full information which rationality in making moral judgements demands.'
>
> (Hare, 1981; p. 92)

Nurse theorists are encouraging and advising practitioners of nursing to put empathy and compassion into their nursing care (Leininger, 1984a; Roach, 1985; Watson, 1990). Thus Scudder, following the logic of Heidegger, suggests that the

> 'authentic nurse would choose a unique way of caring for each particular patient . . . care would be creatively given in response to particular patients for whom the nurse assumes responsibility.'
>
> (Scudder, 1990)

It is the central characteristic of compassion, and in particular empathy, that it is directed towards an individual or specific case. It is not a diffuse generalised state such as pity, where it is possible to have 'pity' on a whole 'class of people', for example the homeless. The emotion is not directed towards any one, specific, homeless young person – rather towards an ill-defined group of 'unknown peoples' who share a particular social-state in common. Should I be concerned with the young homeless man whom I almost fell over, as I left the Underground station? I could be moved by compassion, for compassion can be generated between individuals and certainly in order to feel truly empathetic I would need to consider the individuality of the young man and his life.

Compassion however, and therefore also empathy, carries with it a burden of responsibility. Empathy implies an understanding of the other person, it also implies a responsibility for the knowledge. It is considered unethical to know about another person's sorrow and not to demonstrate concern and care; and perhaps it is the awareness of this phenomenon that is used by those who are suffering to protect the integrity of the would-be carer, as much as to protect themselves from the pains of disclosure and vulnerability. By not allowing the carer to come too close, the patients can protect themselves and the carer; in such cases there is no chance for mutuality, no empathy, no compassion and therefore no responsibility.

It is interesting, as McFarlane notes in her essay on the paradigm of caring in nursing, that the evangelical story of the Good Samaritan portrays him as intervening in the shattered life of the robbed man, because he was 'moved by compassion' and that, having been moved by compassion, he took responsibility for his actions which were thoughtful, deliberate and above all, considerate (McFarlane, 1988).

Empathetic approaches to nursing care are therefore not surprisingly regarded as the key to better caring. Whereas the need for more empathy among nurses may be evident, patient complaints about the falling standards of nursing care appear to be rising. The paradoxical problem remains; how to teach empathy skills and to empathise with patients, when to empathise truly is impossible, and some patients will inevitably provoke the worst feelings in us (Gould; 1990, Holden, 1990; Burnard, 1988). Certainly to empathise and be compassionate one needs to acknowledge a common ground of felt humanity; an acknowledgement of solidarity with the 'broken, fearful and anguished stranger' (Roach, 1985).

To be able to empathise with a patient should not, however, have to depend on our *personal* experiences, but rather on our level of sensitivity and common human understanding of life and life's events. As nurses we should be able to empathise with all patients at least to some degree. The young nursing student who hugs the sobbing mother whose child is being wheeled into surgery is as much empathising with the 'universal-mother-woman' and demonstrating appropriate compassion, as the busy professional nurse consultant in the intensive care unit who tenderly brushes the unconscious patient's hair. Having the time and sensitivity to ensure that the hair does not become matted and full of paste from EEG leads is equally demonstrable of empathy and compassion as is holding an elderly confused patient's hand.

There are many levels of demonstrating compassion and many forms of manifesting care. Unfortunately fine literature abounds with examples where there was no empathy and even less compassion evident. Sometimes the problem lies in the vast socio-cultural gap between care-giver and care-receiver; a problem noted by Leininger in her cross-cultural studies of care phenomena (Leininger, 1978, 1981). Solzenitsyn, in his epic work *Cancer Ward* illustrates this poignantly. Solzenitsyn illustrates how difficult it may be for a health professional to empathise adequately and demonstrate compassion with an adolescent. Asya, a young 18-year-old, has just found out that she has a malignant growth in one of her breasts. She runs to her friend, Dyomka, and breaks down. Of all the horrors awaiting her she can think of only one, that she will not be able to wear a bathing-suit.

'She could never show herself on the beach again. It had suddenly struck her as the most excrutiating, the most mortifying fact of her existence. Living had lost all meaning and this was the reason why.'

(Solzenitsyn, 1969)

Few mature oncology nurses would automatically think of this perceived inability to wear a bathing-suit as the most devastating result of a radical mastectomy for a teenager. To Dyomka, however, her newfound boyfriend, who himself had just lost a leg to the effects of osteogenic sarcoma, this outburst of emotions and its rationale were not strange.

'Dyomka searched for words, but they wouldn't come. All he could do was clasp her hand tighter and tighter to try to stop her. He had *more* pity for her than he had ever had for himself.'

(Solzenitsyn, 1969)

Empathy flourishes where conditions are most like one's own; strangeness on the other hand hinders and prohibits true empathy (Gould, 1990).

If compassion is so heavily dependent on empathy to give it impetus and rationale, then researchers will have to examine more closely those factors that contribute to greater empathy, and also those constructs of caring that can be developed in the absence of initial or naturally occurring empathy. As Gould rightfully points out, one cannot be equally empathetic about all patients; and yet not to recognise this is itself an act of professional un-caring behaviour and certainly not conducive to encouraging a long-term caring approach to patients.

Interestingly where empathy and compassion are seen to be completely lacking, patients often supply each other with this necessary healing power.

Professional empathy, it would appear, is not so much a *personal* projection of affective and cognitive modes of being concerning another, but rather an ability to enter the world of a stranger and attempts to identify with the preferences, loves, and hurts of the other so as to be able effectively to help the other towards the restoration of health and wellbeing.

At some level professional compassion therefore may also be a form of professional companionship (Rawnsley, 1990). Alastair Campbell defines professional companionship as a bodily presence which accompanies the other for a while (Campbell, 1984). As in nursing it may arise from a chance meeting, and the good, effective companion is one who 'shares freely, but does not impose, allowing others to make their own journey' (Campbell, 1984). Thus, perhaps nursing can be seen as a type of journey with patients where the elements of choice and freedom are always present. Empathy as a construct of compassion is seen to be freely given and possessing generative powers. It is not imposed from outside and does not play older sister to pity or even self-contempt, denial or least of all projected protection or paternalism. One of the central characteristics of compassion is that it empowers and promotes freedom and the joy of solidarity with the stranger. This is in contrast to pity, which is a feeling of non-productive sorrow, a wasted grief, for compassion, according to Roach, is a

> 'way of living born out of an awareness of one's relationship to all living creatures. It engenders a response of participation in the experience of another, a sensitivity to the pain and brokenness of the other.'
>
> (Roach, 1985)

Competence

Some nurses may express surprise that in analysing elements of caring behaviours we take time to look at nursing competence. Competence, however, was considered by Roach as one of the five main constructs of caring behaviours. Much has been written recently about nursing competence, especially by nurse educationalists, who desire to establish minimal levels of various nursing skills and competencies, in order to be able to establish adequate educational programmes to meet new learning and practice requirements.

The kind of competence, however, that Roach was referring to is far broader in scope than identifiable behaviours whose sum possession demonstrates attainment of a particular level of nursing expertise. In order to be capable of demonstrating care and caring attitudes as a professional nurse, the nurse must first and foremost be a competent practitioner of nursing.

As Lanara observes, nursing education should promote 'inquiring minds and searching hearts' (Lanara, 1982), and educationalists are rightfully criticised for attempting to educate student-nurses for the profession of nursing according to a task-orientated (checklist of competencies) mentality. If nursing is as broad and all encompassing as Henderson suggests, where:

> ' . . . the nurse is temporarily the consciousness of the uncon-scious, the love of life of the suicidal, the leg of the amputee, the eyes of the newly blind, a means of locomotion for the newborn, knowledge and confidence for the young mother, a voice for those too weak to speak . . . '
>
> (Henderson, 1978)

then the programme preparing young new nurses should reflect this belief. As Henderson (1978) logically concludes:

> 'Nurses, who practise according to this concept, must know how to assess the client's or patient's need for help . . . keep the body clean, warm and clothed . . . they should be masters of their unique role.'
>
> (Henderson, 1978)

It is the mastery of holistic nursing practised by nursing experts that is reflected as professional competence, rather than individual discrete competencies that aggregate to bestow an aura of professionalism on novice nurses. Nurses will demonstrate excellence of practice and professional competence when they have more accountability and authority for their personal practice, and where authority itself comes from extensive knowledge of one's field of concern. Thus Labelle (1978) comments that if nurses had a thorough commitment to on-going learning, which 'includes setting goals and their energetic fulfil-ment, questions of mandatory continuing education would be redun-dant'.

Part of the domain of professional accountability must surely be adequate professional competency to practise. It is precisely because the nurse is a competent practitioner that she is fully accountable for her conduct and is capable of demonstrating a caring approach to her patients and clients.

Again it is Henderson (1980) who notes that:

> ' . . . nurses might more drastically affect the quality of basic nursing if nurses developed the habits and skills of inquiry, if they applied existing research findings and if they thought of "theory" underlying nursing as having no circumscribed limits . . . '
>
> Henderson, 1980)

The presence of an enquiring mind, an appreciation for nursing research, a commitment to implement relevant research findings, and the power and authority to control personal practice, are all indispens-able ingredients making up the persona of the competent caring nurse. Labelle postulates that knowledge of one's field of practice would suggest that ' . . . above all, the nurse would have a prime prerequisite to speaking and behaving with respect and authority' (Labelle, 1978). She recognises, however, that there are at least four factors that affect nursing authority, namely knowledge, accountability, interpersonal relationships and power. According to Labelle (1978) technical and theoretical knowledge (or professional competence) is only a part of the overall equation that needs to be addressed in order for nursing care to be manifest. Rawnsley (1985) points out that:

' . . . Nursing will be defined in history not by its claims, but by its acts. In the existential sense, to do is to be. If we keep our mission in mind – promoting quality of life for our clients through the prevention and amelioration of suffering – then we have a true and lawful goal for our science.'

(Rawnsley, 1985)

In order for the mission of nursing to be clear, and in order for nurses not to lose sight of their goals, they will need to develop theories of nursing and base their practice on sound foundations which will be inculcated into the new recruits to the profession. Ultimately, an increase in professional competence will only occur with a new approach to learning and professional self-development.

Darbyshire would like to see UK nursing education follow Watson's lead, and he would like to base nursing education on a model of nursing where care is the central theme.

'Establishing caring as a founding concept for nurse education is another aim of the curriculum revolution . . . the theme of caring should be a golden thread running through the curriculum.'

(Darbyshire, 1991)

This requires more however, than simply a 'name change and a different set of content in the timetable in order to empower, enthuse and educate students' (Darbyshire, 1991).

A closer investigation of the concept of competency in practice as done by Gaut (1986) and Hutchinson (1990) reveals many interlinking subconstructs such as confidence, authority, responsibility and courage. The areas that may prove most interesting, and fruitful for analysis from an experimental perspective, are the areas of nursing knowledge, and nursing skills acquisition. In order for the nurse to be fully competent and therefore in a position of mastery and control, whatever other professional attributes need to be present, certainly the need to have a sound nursing knowledge base relevant to her area of work and possession of the necessary appropriate skills to function independently will be important. The type, extent and depth of knowledge necessary for nurses to practise is a point of much debate.

Manley (1991) points out that without a theoretical underpinning to our nursing practice it will not be grounded or contained in an analytical structure. It is hard to research, evaluate, promote or even transmit practices and/or values if these are not perceived or formulated in a structured fashion, within an analysable theory. She adds that 'theory' should not curtail practice since it is solely the 'theorists' best efforts to try and describe and explain the phenomena observed' (Manley, 1991; p. 13). Acquisition of knowledge promotes theory formulation, and Manley points out interesting relationships not only between knowledge and theoretical frameworks but the interconnectedness of knowledge and power, knowledge and professionalism, and knowledge and accountability (Manley, 1991).

There is increasing pressure from among leading educationalists to raise the level of academic input in basic nurse education. This move has resulted in the recent re-structuring of nurse education in the United Kingdom, from pre-registration courses through to post-registration nursing degrees. Far more significant than the basic re-structuring of the system of nurse education however, which has profound socio-economic and political effects on the organisation and administration of the National Health Service, is the even greater change that is occurring in the fundamental attitude of nurses to the acquisition and use of nursing knowledge (Manley, 1991).

Apart from such elemental questions as defining what nursing knowledge is, and how acquisition and assimilation of this knowledge may affect nursing practice, we are faced with criticisms. Nursing practice will only be as good as the level of internalisation of care concepts. These are inherent in the various knowledge domains relevant to, and constructing part of that which we call nursing practice. What aspects of knowledge can most adequately help structure nursing practice needs to be researched further.

Toliver (1988) in an interesting article suggests that nursing students (at all levels of study, but especially those preparing for advanced expert practice, such as clinical experts in symptom control or community nursing), should improve their critical thinking skills; a competence which 'is required daily and is, therefore, an expected behaviour of professional nursing' (Toliver, 1988). She notes, like Manley (1991), that declarative and procedural knowledge is important, and adds that:

> ' . . . research indicates that analysis of the elements underlying the inductive reasoning process strengthens learning how to think. With practice and feedback the factual knowledge and the thinking blueprint can become more extensive to novice nurses.'
>
> (Toliver, 1988)

Critical-thinking skills will not 'mechanise' caring structures; rather they will add competence and authority to nursing practice. Powell (1989) also calls for more 'thinking' in nursing, in particular 'reflection-in-action'. She feels that:

> 'Reflection-in-action seems likely to make professional practice more effective, both for present clients/patients and future ones, because of the learning from practice which occurs.'
>
> (Powell, 1989)

Powell sees reflectivity as a matter of degrees or levels, and certainly the ability to think critically and be able to reflect on practice are skills that need to be taught. They do not occur naturally but, as Powell wryly comments, 'an element of questioning and critical thinking certainly facilitates reflection on practice' (Powell, 1989).

Based on empirical evidence of previous omissions in the nursing curriculum, the current attempt to redress the balance, resulting in an emphasis on studies in the humanities and social sciences, seems to be a welcome change. These studies, however, should not be at the expense of the physical and life sciences, which some educationalists argue still form the backbone of nursing concerns (Akinsanya, 1986). The practising nurse can be said most likely to demonstrate clinical caring competence, that is ability to perform sensitive nursing tasks as required by her work, when she *knows* what she should do; that is when she has an adequate nursing *knowledge* and skills base to help her assess, plan and deliver *care*. This knowledge and skills base needs to be informed by a caring passion. As Watson points out:

> ' . . . If knowledge is void of informed passion, it can be used for domination, for manipulation, for control, for power, for fixing the vision for the next generation on a reality others have already predefined.'
>
> (Watson, 1990)

This would be the very opposite of what is the perceived goal and aim of nursing, namely 'the development of a healthy independence' (Henderson, 1978) among patients and clients wherever this is possible. Rawnsley (1985) adds that nurses are 'committed to helping persons move towards wholeness, regardless of the point at which they start'. These aims for nursing would imply an art and science which is inherently empowering and liberating for those whom it serves, as Henderson (1978) emphatically states:

> 'This intimate and essential service is, in my opinion, the universal element in the concept of nursing. It is a *service* . . . '
>
> (Henderson, 1978)

Nurses therefore must be aware of this all embracing imperative, if they truly wish to *serve* their patients, and heed Rawnsley's comment that:

> 'Nursing science must acknowledge those things that can change and those that cannot . . . '
>
> (Rawnsley, 1985)

The assessing, planning and delivering of care involves not only the patient but also the ward or the patient's environment and staff resources. For further ramifications of this process, *see* Chapter 4. It is the nursing knowledge base of the qualified nurse which prompts the practitioner to assess staffing levels, plan staff resources and allocate and designate funds and personnel to particular areas of concern. When this is present, with the commission of adequate nursing skills, then there is an increased likelihood that caring attitudes will be manifested or, at the very least, that structural impediments to the delivery of care have been removed. Lanara states:

> 'Nursing care is care of people on the part of a nurse who understands human beings, their motivations and behaviour. It encompasses planning, administering, and evaluating patient care. Nursing care, therefore, demands continuous exercise of critical thinking, creative imagination, and independent judgement in problem-solving and decision-making.'
>
> (Lanara, 1982)

The issue of levels and types of skills and experience necessary for nurses to function adequately has been addressed by the profession as long ago as the 1960s (Orlando, 1961). The concern now is to admit that, although knowledge may include awareness of nursing skills, there are some forms of knowledge which are predominantly within the spheres of theoretical and conceptual frameworks. It is, however, predominantly a concern for proficiency in technical skills based on informed practice that is perceived as necessary by patients if caring is to be manifested (Forrest, 1989; Geissler, 1990; Cronin and Harrison, 1988). Obviously, as with theoretical knowledge, practical skills can and do encompass all of nursing concerns, and practical skills are as necessary by the bedside or wheelchair as they are in the office, in teaching and in political persuasion. The skill with which a particular action or function is undertaken is as crucial to patient satisfaction and perception of a caring attitude as the knowledge base upon which the practice is grounded (Mayer, 1986; Wolf, 1986; Brown, 1986). However, as Samarel observed concerning the nursing care she received post-operatively:

> 'I needed a combination of auditory, visual, and kinesthetic stimulation for reassurance and reality orientation.'
>
> (Samarel, 1990)

What she sought most was the nurses' caring presence. She adds that:

> ' . . . through personal experience I have learned that nursing must be practised as a caring art if nurses are truly to meet the

psychosocial as well as the physiological needs of their patients.'
(Samarel, 1990)

In practice how does lack of competence hinder a caring attitude? Nursing literature has plenty of examples of nurses who, lacking in 'competence' to do the tasks required of them, could not manifest a caring attitude. Indeed, in some instances they simply could not 'care' (Gould, 1990; Orlando, 1961; Barber, 1991). Sometimes the nurse felt she had a duty of care towards the patient, but was essentially incompetent to deliver that care because of lack of expertise, skills or knowledge-base. Apart from increased anxiety, sometimes leading to withdrawal, patient-labelling, and in extreme cases to professional burn-out, this attitude also leads to ineffective and mechanical delivery of routine care, which is not perceived by the care-receiver as necessarily evidence of 'caring'.

In Simone de Beauvoir's short account of the death of her mother, *A very easy death*, she repeatedly questions the competence of the nurses and physician looking after her mother, since she did not perceive the type of care they gave as particularly 'caring' or effective in relieving distress. At one point the constant moving and shifting of her mother in bed and the changing of sheets, necessitated by the latter's incontinence and an oozing from cancerous wounds, led the two sisters to agree not to change the sheets, even if they were wet, and therefore to spare their mother the pain involved in even the slightest movement (Beauvoir, 1973).

Thirty years on, the development of the hospice movement and the existence of palliative care teams and the considerate nature of district nurses has made this case in some respects, a historical example of bad communication and profound mismatch of goals between the patient and care-givers. Nonetheless, the story is sufficiently horrendous that the novelist-daughter immortalised her dismay at the lack of caring by the health-care team, and in particular nurses, in that very poignant short account of her mother's none-too-easy dying and death at home. If a nurse needs to change a dressing, she should do so as effectively and quickly as possible. The high level of skill necessary to do this task relatively painlessly and efficiently will contribute to a feeling of being competently cared for. An increase in skills and knowledge carries with it a greater awareness of professional accountability for practice and therefore professional responsibility. As Lanara (1982) observed:

'Without the sense of responsibility the nurse cannot carry out nursing in the way people and society demand. A high quality of nursing care presupposes full consciousness of responsibility on the part of the nurse . . . '
(Lanara, 1982)

In the case cited by Beauvoir, there appears to have been minimal professional responsibility for practice. Lanara (1982) continues her observations on responsibility, noting that:

> '. . . true responsibility is dependent upon knowledge, discretion, judgement and the ability to make decisions about one's work.'
> (Lanara, 1982)

It is the latter point that most often obstructs otherwise well prepared and well intentioned nurses. Occasionally even knowledge and skills are lacking.

Not so long ago, in a modern hospital in a metropolitan town in the United Kingdom, a young foreign boy was receiving treatment for burns and having burn dressing changes to massive wounds which he had sustained while pouring petrol on a fire. Every change of dressing was a traumatic event and a focal point for the child's fear and distress. The situation was not helped by a lack of adequate knowledge and skills in the care of burns, from both the medical and nursing teams. It was hard to detect direct 'caring' in that sad, not too unusual case. Lack of adequate *competence* to care for the child led to much needless pain and distress. The situation was 'saved', however, by the limited competence of the nurses in another sphere of operation, which led them to arrange for the child to be transferred to another centre more capable of specialist 'caring'. This case illustrates at least two important points concerning competencies and the extent to which the absence or presence of knowledge and skills contributes to a mutual perception of caring having occurred. Undoubtedly the nurses lacked *specific* knowledge and skills to care adequately for a child with severe burns, but they did possess 'general caring' skills and paediatric nursing knowledge which prompted them to arrange with medical colleagues for the transfer of the child to another centre. It is doubtful that the child perceived this move to another hospital at the time as evidence of caring, and the nurses were left with an overwhelming feeling of inadequacy and guilt. As Gaylin points out:

> 'Guilt and its fellow emotions of caring, loving, shame, compassion, empathy, and pity bind us to those who are needed for our own survival. Guilt may thus be recognised as a guardian of our goodness, calling us back from unhealthy self-absorption to an awareness of the social fabric to which we belong.'
> (Gaylin, 1985; p. 72)

It is clear that in the example some degree of caring was present. Both nursing knowledge and practical nursing skills are necessary for a nurse to practise with competence, but given the complex nature of nursing interventions, the attempt at delivering care may not be immediately evident to the care-receiver or care-giver. Recent research looking at how and when patients perceive caring to occur would appear to suggest, at this early, preliminary stage, that the more acutely ill a patient is, not surprisingly the more significance they attach to physical and technical manifestations of caring, while nurses tend to down-grade this sphere of activity (Cronin and Harrison, 1988; Morrison, 1989; Forrest, 1989).

Paul Barber, in his provocative chapter on caring in *Nursing: A Knowledge Base for Practice*, observes that he would have appreciated *both* theoretical and practical skills to be present among the nurses who cared for him. Technical competence is extremely important, but this must be grounded in relevant nursing theory and always accompanied by critical analysis and continuous reflection on the efficacy of practice (Barber, 1991).

Undoubtedly it is more difficult to care spiritually and psychologically for patients than to develop expertise in a technical area of care. Moments of truly integrated, holistic caring are like precious jewels, difficult to attain but beautiful when they are found. Nonetheless, it is part of the power of professional insight and empathy to understand when technical expertise is needed in addition to psycho-social skills. Often it is expertise in both domains that is required, and caring is most likely to occur when the balance of psycho-social, spiritual, and technical expertise is felt to be just right. Orlando, in the early 1960s, beautifully illustrated cases where nursing with sensitivity, empathy and technical skills, plus a sound knowledge base, all worked together to provide instances of caring for distraught, angry or mis-understood patients (Orlando, 1961). This technique of teaching caring skills by drawing attention to moments and instances of 'true caring' is an approach used by several writers and nurse-theorists, most recently Benner (1984) and Benner and Wrubel (1989). As Watson (1990) observes:

'. . . we do not and cannot create nursing and caring knowledge in a void . . . My plea is for informed passion, passion that is informed by thought, reflection and contemplation, giving rise to moral landscapes and contexts of human and mature relational concerns.'

(Watson, 1990)

Finally, as Roach defines competence, it is the 'state of having the knowledge, skills, energy, experience, and motivation required to respond adequately to the demands of one's professional responsibilities' (Roach, 1985). Campbell additionally observes that to be professional is to 'show the ability and willingness to develop one's talents in the service of others' (Campbell, 1985). Professionalism demands competence, and in turn sustains rightful power and authority to implement effective caring practice, for:

> 'While competence without compassion can be brutal and inhumane, compassion without competence may be no more than a meaningless, if not harmful, intrusion into the life of a person or persons needing help.'
>
> (Roach, 1985)

Confidence

Confidence is rarely thought of as a subconstruct of caring. Indeed, there is at least one image of the caring nurse where she appears, superficially to be quiet, gentle and almost timorous. It is possible that this particular portrait of the caring nurse owes its origin to the mistaken notion that quietness and gentleness, (which may *almost* verge on timidity) are present in caring nurses. So often nurses that care are indeed gentle and quiet, and appear to approach the patient or client with an air of apology for intruding into the patient's private world. Confidence, however, should also never be associated with boisterousness or a notion of being opinionated. Neither should assertiveness be confused with aggressiveness and anger. To possess and to exude confidence can only be manifested if the nurse is in control of her nursing domain; and if the nurse is empowered with authority and responsibility to nurse to the best of her ability.

Levine, in one of her early works, comments on the need for the 'ethics of competence and the ethics of compassion' to regulate and guide clinical accountability. It is impossible, she argues, to talk of moral professional conduct without acknowledging the roles that clinical competence, and professional compassion play in the determinants of morally viable accountable practice (Levine, 1977).

Bergman (1981), in her position paper on nursing accountability, eloquently points out that accountability contains within its central definition three core concepts: 1) personal responsibility, 2) the nature of authority and 3) the need for reporting back. Where most nurse theoreticians would acknowledge that personal responsibility is a key component of accountability, Bergman actually visualises accountability as being the apex of a complex moral-identity triangle with ability, knowledge, skills and values at the base. The practitioner of nursing moves through phases of responsibility and authority in order to be held ultimately accountable, and to be in a position of accountability (Bergman, 1981). It is the totally accountable nurse, exercising professional accountability for informed practice, who promotes confidence in herself, her profession and the health-care system. It is in such a nurse that the patient can place his trust.

There are two main sub-constructs of confidence: confidence which the nurse exudes and is therefore controlled from the nurse's own psychic-centre; and confidence which the patient places in the nurse. The nurse exudes confidence because she has sufficient knowledge, skills and authority to implement her plan of care. She is also confident in herself and her profession. Perfect confidence can only come as a result of deep self-awareness and self-acceptance, warts and all, and a deliberate attempt at continual self-growth. Nursing, as an interpersonal art requires many skills that call for tempered self-disclosure, which in turn requires much self-awareness; to be comfortable with oneself is not easy, and it is this personal comfortableness that is perceived by 'the other' as confidence.

In a fascinating account of professional 'responsible subversiveness', Hutchinson eloquently demonstrates the level of professional and personal moral integrity required to have the courage to carry through that level of care necessary to maintain trust with the patient (Hutchinson, 1990). According to Hutchinson, the level of care required to maintain trust may call for subversion; courageous, deliberate transgressions of rules, regulations and 'common-practice'. Rule-breaking and bending is not done lightly but, in her fascinating study, it was the clinical 'experts' who saw the need to violate rules in order to maintain patient confidence, often at enormous psychological cost to themselves, and at the risk of losing their professional work. As she wryly comments, 'responsible subversion is a complex process that requires energy and effort; following rules is inevitably easier' (Hutchinson, 1990).

The second type of confidence concerns that which is entrusted in the nurse. It is the caring nurse who encourages the patient to place himself 'in her confidence', that is, in her trust. The patient is not always aware of why he feels he 'trusts' a certain nurse, why he feels confident that a particular nurse will 'care' for him, and even less often is he capable of verbalising his innermost thoughts concerning confiding in a particular nurse and knowing that his confidence will be vindicated. Just as the patient commits himself to potential rejection and hurt, so does the nurse. As in all aspects of the possibility of caring, the potential for hurt and rejection is always there. Entrusting a nurse with his confidence can make the patient, at least temporarily, appear quite vulnerable. Examples of the presence of confidence and trust as a sub-construct of caring in the popular, non-professional literature are few, but those that do exist are very eloquent. Perhaps one of the most moving is the story told by Antoine de Saint-Exupery. In the 1930s Saint-Exupery worked for the pioneering mail-courier service between Europe and countries of Latin America. During one such flight over the Andes, a small aeroplane crashed on the snows and the pilot-mailman, one of his friends, found himself stranded in the high valleys of the Chilean mountains. A search for the airman, Guillaumet, was organised and for several days his colleagues flew over the valleys, looking for their friend. Eventually the search was called off, but Saint-Exupery continued the search, flying dangerously low and well beyond any 'reasonable' period of viable survival for his friend. The friend, however, miraculously survived and lived to tell the tale of how he *knew* that Saint-Exupery would search for him. He was completely *confident* that search parties would be organised, led by his ace-pilot friend, Antoine, and he recalled how he knew even which plane was Saint-Exupery's. 'You see', he said,

> 'no-one would continue searching so long after the accident and no-one else would fly so low in the valleys between the craggy mountains, at risk of their own life, but you. Just knowing it was you, reaffirmed my *confidence* in you; I knew *you* cared; I had the energy to continue climbing on, even though you could not see me, I could see you.'

> (Saint-Exupery, 1972)

This example from literature can find an echo in much of the work of our front line rescue workers such as life-boat workers, alpine-patrol skiers or ambulance workers. The same is often said about nurses. To have confidence in someone, implies entrusting them with that which we hold valuable, e.g. our health, our lives, our children, or even our tasks and petitions.

Meize-Grochowski (1984) in an excellent analysis of the concept of trust as it applies to nurses in their daily work, observes that trust consists of at least five component parts which she defines as (1) attitude, (2) reliability, (3) confidence, (4) time and space binding and (5) fragility. She defines trust as an attitude 'bound to time and space in which one relies with confidence on someone or something. Trust is further characterized by its fragility' (Meize-Grochowski, 1984). Furthermore, supporting her argument with case illustrations, she explains what she considers to be the antecedents of trust, among which she lists consistent behaviour or action of someone, or a positive experience in the past, in relation to someone or something (Meize-Grochowski, 1984). Interestingly, she too, like Hutchinson (1990), notes that trust involves 'an element of risk in past association of a person with someone or something'. As to the consequences of trust, that is, the results of positive trusting, she identifies the following:

i   a sharing of feelings between two persons
ii development of a therapeutic relationship

iii an openness and honesty between two persons
iv a reinforcement of trust in someone or something.

Meize-Grochowski's work needs to be continued and expanded if modern nurses analysing attributes of caring are to command adequate academic and professional respect.

Pepper, writing about cancer nurses, calls this quality of being able to give patients confidence and ability to impart hope, an integral aspect of 'caring' (Pepper, 1985). Pepper, echoing Meize-Grochowski's comments concerning the fragility of trust and how easily it is broken, quotes a young oncology nurse stating her philosophy of care. It is in keeping with Pepper's own philosophy of a trinity of care, love and hope, which he claims needs to be made manifest to the patients:

> 'You have this unusual involvement to begin with, and sometimes it gets deeper, more complex than it should. Because the more vulnerable they are, the closer you come to them.'
>
> (Pepper, 1985)

Nurses can confirm the patient's estimation that the nurse is caring for them not only because they encourage patients to hope, but, most importantly, they encourage patients to have faith and confidence in themselves. This confidence is evident by the diligent persistence of the nurses in performing duties, almost, in the patient's perception, above and beyond the call of duty.

Beverly Hall (1990), in an article analysing the constructs of hope among AIDS patients, sensitively demonstrates how a nurse who exudes confidence can impart hope; and how these patients can radically alter their approach to life, death, and the disease process, because they trust their nurses and physicians. They have confidence in the health-care system and feel empowered with hope to challenge the negative aspects of the disease process. In order to be able to share this amount of life-restoring energy and hope, the nurses themselves must have authority over their practice, be expert practitioners and be accountable to their professional body and their patients. She notes that among other attributes, possessing hope 'involves finding a treatment in the professional or alternative care system that one believes will contribute to survival' (Hall, 1990). Such 'faith' in a treatment plan involves confidence in the system, and often it is nurses who can show bewildered patients the way forward, or who can demonstrate faith and hope in humanity when it would appear that such faith is fruitless. These examples are often highly visible in times of war and distress, e.g., midwives delivering babies in Nazi concentration camps, or nurses crossing no-man's land to tend the wounds of soldiers on both sides of the barricades. But what of the staff nurses who inspire confidence in patients and relatives in the small hours of the morning on busy surgical wards? This occurs when the patient feels that he can rely on the nurse to keep his family informed of his condition, and he knows he will not be let down. The nurse is poised and self-assured; she has authority, and she attracts the goodwill of her colleagues as much as she encourages trust from her patients.

This essential ingredient in the ability to care, the ability to encourage confidence in nursing practice, as with all the caring sub-constructs, is very fragile (Meize-Grochowski, 1984). How often, unfortunately, we hear patients say that they have no confidence in the ability of the nurse, due to the latter's lack of adequate skills, expertise, knowledge or even authority to carry through necessary nursing care. It is hard to perceive caring behaviours or intent in nurses who say one thing but do something else; who assures the patient that their post-operative pain will be adequately controlled, but neglect the needs of the post-operative patient and do not hear what the patient has to say (Barber, 1991). In order for the patient to have confidence in his care-giver, he must *see and feel* care being delivered. He must be assured that the nurse is aware of the patient's condition. Confidence, it would appear, relies heavily on the nurse's personal integrity and ability to build and maintain trust (Meize-Grochowski, 1984).

Nelda Samarel, a professor of nursing, in an interesting account of her own personal experiences in a recovery-room following a thyroidectomy, confirms the observation that in order for the patient to have confidence in the nurse and to feel 'cared for', the nurse needs to be not only competent by professional standards, but *appear* to be competent to the patient. She needs to be seen, felt, and heard to be concerned with and about the state of the patient. She comments that personalising the care would have gone a long way to allaying her fears:

> 'The nurse continually tried to reassure me by saying, "The operation is over. You're in the recovery room". Yet those words offered me no reassurance. I was not sure they were directed to me . . . I questioned the reality of the words as I questioned the reality of my entire experience. Perhaps the words would have seemed more real if I heard my name.'
>
> (Samarel, 1990)

The writer notes that she knew she was cared for when she felt and saw the nurse; otherwise, even though the nurse was there, as a patient she had no confidence in her. She needed constant visual and tactile contact with the nurse for re-assurance. Thus she continues:

'What was reassuring was being touched . . . When I felt the nurse's touch, *I knew* she was present and *I knew* she was taking care of me . . .'

(Samarel, 1990)

This experience is similar to Barber's (1991) experience. He additionally noted that the situation is rendered even more difficult to remedy when the nurses are not perceived to be even marginally competent. He notes that they did not adequately assess his pain, they fabricated a patient scenario that was not there . . . No wonder he felt that his care was inadequate. He had little confidence in the nurses, and the nurses did little to promote an aura of confidence about themselves. He felt bereft of *professional* help and was left entirely to his own inner strengths for the energy to survive, heal and recuperate. It is interesting that the turning point in his healing process occurred after his wife expertly delivered a massage of his back. The combination of muscle relaxation, increased blood circulation, and the psychospiritual healing resulting from close intentional therapeutic touching, renewed *confidence* in himself and those close to him, which resulted in a definite turning point in the healing process. The massage contributed to the renewal of his confidence in himself, his inner resources, the power and strength of his wife, and the healing presence of his family. It is notable that the nurses concerned with his care did not offer a massage, indeed very few modern nurses ever offer to give patients back-rubs. This is often due to lack of time, but possibly more significantly due to lack of motivation, lack of knowledge of the physiological benefits of massage, and minimal understanding of the multiple, psycho-spiritual benefits that intentional touch can stimulate. For further ramifications on alternative therapies see Chapter 5.

Certainly Dr Barber had little confidence in the system, even less in the nursing staff, and any confidence he managed to tap was generated by his wife and family. As Samarel concludes:

'What I sought, to meet my needs during this most stressful event, was the nurse's caring presence . . . Caring denotes concern, devotion and commitment and is expressed non-verbally more than verbally . . . Her visual presence and her touch conveyed a caring that comforted me.'   (Samarel, 1990)

This, it could be added, exuded professionalism and confidence, which carries its own therapeutic message. Confidence in themselves and the nursing staff was missing as much for Samarel as it was for Barber.

In conclusion Roach defines nursing confidence as:

'that quality which fosters trusting relationships . . . confidence which fosters trust without dependency, communicates truth without violence . . . which creates respect without paternalism and ensures a relationship which does not compromise the freedom and independence of clients by rendering them powerless.'

(Roach, 1985)

Conscience

When looking at constructs of caring, one area that is often referred to but not elaborated upon, and implied but rarely analysed, is the level of moral integrity required of the practising nurse. Traditionally, when referring to the moral domain and its imperatives, the leaders of nursing would write about the nurse's conscience as a connation of professional and personal values, so internalised by the practitioner that she practised her art according to a particular pre-set moral blueprint laid down by the pioneers of the profession. This left little room for individual moral growth or variation.

According to Roach (1985) conscience, as a construct of caring and one of her five elements of caring behaviour, is defined as a 'sensitive, informed sense of what is right and wrong, a compass directing one's behaviour according to prescribed moral standards' (Roach, 1985). Recently however, to talk of having a conscience, personal or professional, has been considered not particularly fashionable, and yet increasingly, moral developmentalists, social psychologists, moral theologians and ethicists and nurse theoreticians are returning to the difficult task of defining 'conscience'; analysing its structures and premises contained in its definition, and attempting to demonstrate how an informed professional and personal conscience may direct practice, shape decisions and affect behaviour (Griffin, 1983; Carper, 1979; Fry, 1989; Watson, 1990).

The traditional nurse's conscience consisted in part of a professional internalisation of Victorian work values, and in part of a carefully fostered Judaeo-Christian 'Western' approach to a particular kind of gestalt and world-view. The professional internalisation of work values is as much in evidence today as it was 50 or 100 years ago (Jolley, 1989). This discussion, however, concerns more than just professional moral integrity, such as maintaining professional confidentiality or behaving in an essentially truthful manner, such as telling patients the truth. Virtues can be and indeed need to be practised outside of professional nursing; for they are practised in addition to professional 'virtues', such as those considered specific to the nature of nursing work. Virtues need to be cultivated not only on a professional level, but also on a personal level, because their cultivation helps mould and develop the personality of an individual. In turn a person's individuality is supported by the fostering of a virtuous life, according to Aristotle. Additionally, fostering a virtuous life predisposes us to viewing incidents in our lives in a specific way, as Hauerwas (1985) notes:

> 'As persons of character we do not confront situations as mud puddles, into which we have to step; rather, the kind of "situations" we confront and how we understand them are a function of the kind of people we are . . . To be a person of virtue therefore involves acquiring the linguistic, emotional, and rational skills that give us the strength to make our decisions and our life our own.'
>
> (Hauerwas, 1985; p. 120)

It is the empowerment to see and to act that stems from the cultivation of personal virtue that is of interest to us professionally.

Some virtues specific to the world of nursing may be considered those that overlap with a particular form of work ethos which are deeply embedded in the Victorian image of the subservient nurse-cum-paid-companion (Jolley, 1989). Even today, arriving on time to work for an early shift is seen more as a moral attribute necessary in the 'good nurse' than as a pragmatic approach to the smooth administration of the ward (which may indeed, coincidentally, demonstrate that the nurse *cares* about her colleagues and the patients on the ward). This approach is evidenced by the fact that such persistent or even excessive punctuality is often perceived as virtuous and worthy of comment on recommendations and job appraisal forms. Interestingly, staying longer and working overtime is often not commented upon at all. The staff nurse who 'willingly' works overtime, double shifts and 'simply leaves late' is acknowledged privately as being 'dedicated' to her work; a moral characteristic worthy of praise, but this is not formalised in the way punctuality may be. This is because it is felt that nurses should love their work and care enough about their hospital to make personal sacrifices to help out in times of pressure or crises. Such are the unwritten premises of the nursing ethos. Transgressions of these professional work statutes evoke not only hierarchical disdain, but, in some instances, administrative wrath and even emotional blackmail, such as the admonition that, 'If you don't work that extra shift, no one will be available to cover for our patients'. More significantly, the nurse who breaks such premises herself feels unworthy of her profession and profoundly guilty. It is the presence of these affective modes of lowered self-esteem and guilt that project these otherwise work-related issues into the arena of moral discord and concern.

Gaylin considered aspects of 'guilt' and 'conscience' significant enough in the constructs of caring theory that he wrote a whole chapter on the nature and essence of 'conscience' in his book on *Caring* (Gaylin, 1976). Like Roach (1985) he felt that aspects of moral integrity are of fundamental relevance to the nature of caring. Gaylin sees conscience as the 'homoncular foreign body abrasively occupying our inner spaces, an irritant for good' (Gaylin, 1976). However, Gaylin additionally sees at least two separate frames of reference when it comes to defining 'guilt', which in turn is the activator of our conscience. One is a focus on guilt that Gaylin calls 'guilty fear' which he describes as a fear which quickly leads to elation and relief

> 'when the footsteps at the door at the moment our hand is in the cookie jar turn out to be those of a younger brother; or when the whizzing siren goes past us and apprehends the 'perpetrator' in the car ahead of us.'
>
> (Gaylin, 1976)

This guilty fear is closely connected with a sense of well-deserved punishment,

> ' . . . it is the awareness that we are about to have something unpleasant inflicted on us which, however, we deserve.'
>
> (Gaylin, 1976)

A true sense of guilt, according to Gaylin, 'does not stand or fall on impending punishment'. It is directed from within ourselves, not from without. Indeed, as Gaylin observes, true guilt is usually at its worst when there is no punishment entailed; it is relieved at the possibility of punishment. True guilt is an indicator of the level of self-criticism or appraisal, since it is not a fear of punishment. In fact it is not fear at all, but rather a specific type of disappointment in self; it is the comparison of 'is' and 'ought' that is at the heart of ethical reasoning (Gaylin, 1976). It is precisely because true guilt is such a powerful motivator towards self-actualisation that it is considered integral to moral behaviour; and caring is defined as a particular form of moral behaviour, since:

> 'the crucial linkage lies in understanding that moral behaviour and conscience are directly related to the process of identification.'
>
> (Gaylin, 1976)

Thus it is that nurses, failing to reach internalised standards, yet attempting to be an idealised image of the 'Perfect Carer', feel guilty and their professional conscience is activated; they feel they have betrayed themselves and their patients. It is well to remember, however, that as Gaylin notes:

> 'both acts of conscience, [i.e. guilty fear and true guilt] enter into unselfish behaviour and acts of kindness and into that which is

lumped together as "caring", but they are different mechanisms, enhanced or diminished by a different set of experiences.'

(Gaylin, 1976)

The nurse feels guilty and experiences moral distress because she is faced with morally unequal demands on her time, energy and personal resources. The nurse's professional conscience is unquiet, and left unattended can lead to all the symptoms and manifestations of professional burn-out; namely apathy, passive anger, non-attendance at work, callous and distancing approaches to patients and colleagues, and in the final and most extreme cases, abandoning nursing altogether (Gould, 1990; Kramer, 1976). The professional conscience is fostered by the nursing profession itself.

Much of the writing on the function of the conscience in the 'caring' literature focuses on the nurse's conscience and this is understandable since it is seen as an integral component of her caring behaviour and certainly considered by Roach to be one of the five elements of caring behaviour. The possession of a conscience is not limited however, solely to nurses and Landingham, in demonstrating the applicability of Roy's model of nursing to patient care, (especially for those who are suffering various forms of guilt, directly or indirectly related to their disease), has written an interesting chapter on the need for nurses to recognise various forms of guilt, and the importance of identifying guilt and guilty behaviour in patients if we are to serve and care for them fully (Van Landingham, 1984; p. 376). The importance of guilt as a potential force for positive or negative change stems from the belief that a person

'develops, changes, and redefines his or her concept of self in response to growth, challenge and crisis. The adapting person is constantly confronted with needs, oughts, and possibilities.'

(Van Landingham, 1984; p. 377)

The problem with faulty guilt and with a non-productive conscience, is that, as Van Landingham (1984) notes when the person experiences guilt:

'his or her self-concept is threatened or disrupted, thereby lowering self-esteem and causing a reduction in coping energy.'

Faulty, non-productive guilt and a non-empowering conscience need to be identified early by the nurse during the assessment phase of interaction and the necessary intervention can then be applied, in order to restore equilibrium and facilitate a trusting relationship as well as to promote caring. Guilt, however, is one of the more personal of emotions; it can be difficult to interpret (Gaylin, 1985; p. 67), and yet its presence can be very disquieting. As Gaylin observes, it is as if our internal structure were torn apart. Gaylin is quite emphatic in stating that the presence of true guilt is an essential human quality:

> 'The failure to feel guilt is the basic flaw of the psychopath, or antisocial person, who is capable of committing crimes of the vilest sort without remorse or contrition.'
>
> (Gaylin, 1985; p. 62)

The nursing profession has two main and unfortunately sometimes opposing forces within it, namely, the educative and the clinical branches, and both these forces play vital roles in shaping and developing the nurse's conscience (Jolley, 1989). It has been observed that the interplay and discordance between the moral imperatives stressed by nursing educationalists and nursing practitioners, itself is the cause of much moral disquiet and unease. Kramer's classic description of the extent of disillusionment experienced by novice nurses when faced with the realities of the nursing world bears out the assumption that part of the moral distress felt by nurses is generated intra-professionally and this is not a helpful ingredient in the formation of a sound and healthy nursing conscience. The other main contribution to the formation of the nurse's conscience is the nurse's own personal value system. A personal value system may include a highly structured approach to morality and a spiritual emphasis that subscribes to a particular form of religious expression and/or an individually processed moral stance which is a thought-through personal moral approach and opinion on life, life-events and the world around us.

Personal conscience plays a significant role in formulating a caring mode, especially in drawing attention to neglect and/or transgressions against another. Thus Mayeroff, in his book on *Caring* notes that the function of a conscience is to tell one ' . . . that something is wrong; if it is felt deeply, understood, and accepted, it provides me with the opportunity to return to my responsibility for the other' (Mayeroff, 1971; p. 35). This almost 'educative' role of the conscience is confirmed when Mayeroff elaborates on the inter-connectedness of caring modes and moral integrity, saying, that one does not 'resume caring to overcome guilt, but overcomes guilt by renewed caring'.

Renewed caring is necessary whenever normal caring patterns have been broken, and the vigilant conscience reacts and guilt sets in. Renewed caring in such instances is necessary not only to restore the balance of interpersonal relationships but also to help to start rebuilding the shattered integrity of the individual, for, according to Mayeroff, through our caring we 'identify with the growth of the other, and experience it as in some sense an extension of myself, my neglect of it produces at the same time a break in my own responsiveness to myself' (Mayeroff, 1971; p. 35). Therefore, he deduces logically that 'guilt in caring is not simply an expression of my betrayal of the other; it is also an expression of self-betrayal' (Mayeroff, 1971; p. 35). Mayeroff also notes an interesting phenomena. Once trust has been broken, and guilt sets in, our conscience awakens and we choose to renew our caring mode. The situation, however, is no longer the same as it was prior to the uncaring incident. The situation is one where patient and nurse are both aware of the fragility of the situation, as Mayeroff points out:

'Return does not necessarily reinstate the relationship as it existed prior to the break; rather, it often makes for a deeper seriousness and awareness of my trust.'

(Mayeroff, 1971; p. 35)

The 'personal' conscience of the nurse plays at least as important a role in the formation of the nurse's professional conscience as does the professional ethos; the latter often embedded in a professional code of conduct. As nursing professionals, educationalists and behaviourists started to look at how children and young people develop morally and form moral judgements, several interesting facts became evident. Van Hooft (1990) observed:

'If the motivational force to act well requires reflection on previous actions along with well-formed attitudes, then how does one get started on the path to ethical living?'

(Van Hooft, 1990)

Ultimately, the cultivation of virtue and moral integrity is dependent on moral education, the formation and cultural integration or, even in the context of a profession, the socialisation of an individual into the unconscious practice of certain habits.

The personal, in contrast to professional, moral development of today's young person probably follows established lines of sequential social and psychological development, as noted by Erickson (1963), Piaget (1932) and Kohlberg (1986). American nurse-theorists and moral developmentalists looking at the moral development of nurses and women acknowledge that they too follow a specific pattern of sequencing of moral sophistication and decision-making (Noddings 1984; Gilligan, 1982).

The most celebrated and for some, notorious modern moral developmentalist is Lawrence Kohlberg and several nurse theorists acknowledge his influence on their work. Kohlberg saw moral development as occurring in circumscribed stages, following the pioneering work of Piaget and Erickson (Piaget, 1932; Erickson, 1963). Nurses living in a westernised society, into which they are successfully integrated, will most likely appear to have reached a particular level of moral development equating to stages four or five of Kohlberg's Moral

Development Scale (Kohlberg, 1986). Few individuals entering the profession of nursing or even during their working life will ever reach stage 6 of Kohlberg's Moral Development Scale, which others have equated with Maslow's final stages of developmental needs (Maslow, 1970). This final stage is reached only by a few self-actualised individuals. The concern that is secondary to this issue, and a raging debate, is on levels of moral functioning and reasoning; but it is central to notions of a nurse's conscience, as is the question 'How does the nurse reconcile the admonitions of her profession as if she had reached stage 6 of Kohlberg's Moral Development Scale, while in reality, on a personal and therefore at a morally far more intimate level, she simply does not function at that stage or in that manner.' Not only is there an inbuilt cause for distress and disquiet, but there is also the problem that a nurse may display stage 6 reasoning professionally in a clinical situation, but on a personal level act according to a far less emotionally or spiritually taxing code of conduct; an observation borne out in much of the criticisms of Kohlberg's work and noted by ethicists, especially Noddings (1984) and Gilligan (1982).

This example can also be easily reversed, and there is a dearth of evidence of apparently mismatched professional and personal value systems, sufficient that Kohlberg had to acquiesce to the just criticism that one can 'know' what should be done, e.g., in a professional context, but not implement this moral knowledge in practice. This point was not picked up in his original research, and even more significantly, because the nurse and health-care professional are additionally bound by a code of conduct, (an additional professional conscience), in the clinical area a nurse may appear far more 'virtuous' superficially or indeed behave so *de facto*, than she might in private life.

This is a situation that even the Greek philosophers had not thought through. If an individual is capable of higher moral reasoning, it was assumed that moral conduct in private and public life would mirror this. The death of Socrates remains the silent witness to this conviction. These issues require far more analysis and research than has hitherto been the case, for not the least of reasons that one of the five main constructs of caring is the nurse's personal moral input. Her level of moral integrity, which is regulated and developed by her personal and professional values, needs to be clearly identified and described and any glaring impediments to the smooth integration of these personal and professional values, removed or modified. Caring can be illustrated when moral integrity is present. Likewise moral disintegration, absence of clear moral aims or purpose or simply moral distress due to a variety of reasons, may be negatively reflected in professional caring contexts. Thus the nurse, who in spite of her personal preferences and aesthetic values can empathetically take care of the patient with a disfiguring ailment, or the nurse who can put aside personal religious inclinations sufficiently to nurse with humane compassion the patient with syphilis or AIDS, is an example of someone for whom professional moral directives and personal human moral develop-ment, irrespective of specific religious tradition is sufficiently well-developed to direct everyday practice in a positive manner. Examples of heroic practice abound. Perhaps the very nature of nursing encour-ages a particular type of person with a particular form of moral integrity to enlist in the profession, though this is probably unlikely. It is however, a comfortable suggestion, but one still needing much research and analysis. Far more common is the nurse who finds the integration of personal and professional norms a problem; the nurse who is not particularly reflective and not particularly inclined to analyse her moral precepts, partly because she has no guidance and partly because up until now this has been a neglected area of profes-sional concern. The conscience of such a nurse is sufficient for every-day working purposes and conforms comfortably with Kohlberg's lower stages of moral development. Hare, stating the obvious ob-serves: 'Our common intuitions are sound ones, if they are, just because they yield acceptable precepts in common cases' (Hare, 1981; p. 49). Given that the majority of the human race also functions at these levels (per definition), is it appropriate that the nursing profes-sion demands of its practitioners the attainment of the dizzy heights of Kohlberg's Moral Development stages 5 and 6, where complete personal autonomy and accountability for personal and professional acts are reflected in reflexive moral behaviour, conducive to a truly caring milieu? Few developmentalists would suggest that helping professions only recruit members who have reached the higher levels of needs attainment, (as per Maslow's Theory of Development) or those who have reached Kohlberg's level 5 and 6 of moral develop-ment, and yet the professions themselves put almost unattainable goals as an example of perfect practice (Gould, 1990).

Hare, continuing with his line of thought that general acceptance of moral precepts may be socially advantageous (and therefore in a professional context, worth isolating, analysing and if need be incor-porating into a code of conduct), adds that 'it is highly desirable that we should all have these intuitions and that our conscience should give us a bad time if we go against them' (Hare, 1981).

Some philosophers would suggest that to aid the individual in developing a 'conscience', critical thinking may help, thus, according to Hare,

> 'critical thinking aims to select the best set of prima facie principles (of moral conduct) for use in intuitive thinking . . . such employ-ment may lead to the improvement of the principles themselves, but it need not; a principle may be overridden without being altered. The best set (of principles, based on critical thinking) are

those whose acceptance yields actions, dispositions, etc. most
nearly approximating to those which would be chosen if we were
able to use critical thinking all the time.'

(Hare, 1981; p. 50)

This is good news for nurses, who claim that they 'think on their feet',
have little time for ethical reflections and yet are faced with issues
related to the quality and integral nature of their caring, all the time.
Most nurses behave in a morally intuitive manner, and analysis of their
actions would probably reveal little difference between a critical
thinking approach, that is a reflexive approach and their ad hoc
intuitive thinking. There is one problem, however, and that is that
besides ordering the priority of selected principles for analysis, critical
thinking is employed for the purpose of aiding in the resolution of
conflicts and in cases of moral uncertainty. Intuitive thinking here, if it
is not based on reflexive practices, may not be very helpful, as:

'those who insist that there can be conflicts of duties are quite right
as regards the intuitive level; for there can indeed be conflicts of
duties which are irresolvable *at that level*, and they can cause all the
anguish that anybody desires.'

(Hare, 1981; p. 53)

As one of the five main constructs of caring, the presence of a nursing
conscience is both a contentious supposition, and an ambiguous term
that begs tighter definition and further clarification. It is clear,
however, that a certain level of moral development and integrity (yet
to be defined) is necessary for the total integration of personal and
professional value norms. When these are present in near perfect
equilibrium, then at least a base is prepared from which caring
attributes can spring. It would be difficult to imagine caring as being
present where moral integration is absent, since, as Roach points out:

'the nurse who "cares" sees the development of a refined, informed, moral conscience no longer *an option*, but a professional
responsibility.'

(Roach, 1985, emphasis mine)

Commitment

There is a form of caring, indeed some would argue a basic component
of caring, that assumes a certain degree of commitment by the care-
giver to the care-receiver (Roach, 1985). The commitment that the
care-giver needs in order to demonstrate optimally her ability and
desire to care, is commitment above all to the patient, that she, the

nurse, *will care*, and that she will undertake to look out for the best interests of her patients. The caring commitment involves a form of promise or pledge; a professional assurance that the nurse will engage herself in the interests of the patient. According to Roach (1985), commitment is a

> 'quality of investment of self in a task, a person, choice or a career, a quality which becomes so internalised as a value that what one is obliged to do is not regarded as a burden.'

This particular construct of caring comes closest to examining the notion of fidelity, professional and interpersonal, within the context of caring.

To promise to engage oneself on behalf of the patient, to be concerned with the inner world of the patient sufficiently and consistently enough to reassure the patient or client that their concerns are important and their needs will be addressed for as long as is necessary; this pledge is at the heart of nursing. Inherent somewhere in the idea of commitment is the notion of long-lasting faithfulness. Commitment is not a passing phenomena or emotion or manifestation of a moral virtue which we only have while the patient is present and 'in our care'. Commitment primarily addresses that aspect of caring which accepts timelessness as an integral element, indeed a vital part of the moral obligation. Thus, once a commitment is made to care for another, time and to some extent effort become immaterial.

It is Saint-Exupery who explains so naturally the timelessness and boundlessness of commitment. In his book *Southern Mail* he described a unique level of commitment to a colleague of his; an internalised commitment of faithfulness which was experienced so strongly that it ultimately galvanised the pilot to continue to struggle for survival, because he, the crashed pilot, knew that others were *committed* to him. He *knew* they believed in him, and they in turn assumed that he would go on. Commitment certainly has the power of motivating the other party, to fulfilling their part of the covenant relationship. It is a mutually binding covenant. The fostering of mutuality and the formation of contractual relationships is not accidental however. Saint-Exupery would say

> ' . . . human relations must be created. One must go through an apprenticeship to learn the job . . . When we exchange manly handshakes, compete in races, join together to save one of us who is in trouble, cry aloud for help in the hour of danger – only then do we learn that we are not alone on earth.'
>
> (Saint-Exupery, 1967)

Thus, according to Saint-Exupery, in order to feel part of a relationship one must deliberately foster a sense of belonging to another, a sense of conscious concern with another, otherwise there will be no possibility for mutuality, not to mention a therapeutic relationship.

The rationale behind fostering a sense of commitment is that one is committed to a patient in order to promote growth via a *caring* relationship. In the nursing context commitment to the patient is part of the moral contract that the nurse undertakes, when caring for her patient (Cooper, 1990; Darbyshire, 1990; Liehr, 1989; Rawnsley, 1990). It is interesting to note that in Leo Tolstoy's awesome short story, *The Death of Ivan Ilych*, it is the faithful servant Gerasim who nurses his master most consistently and with true commitment. Friends, family and the medical profession all colluded against Ivan Ilych, but the dogged faithfulness of Gerasim, who listened and fulfilled his master's wishes and committed himself to his master's needs provided the only moments of relief the poor man received during the last weeks and days of his life. Ivan Ilych discovered that:

> 'Gerasim did it all easily, willingly, simply, and with a good nature that touched Ivan Ilych. Health, strength and vitality in other people were offensive to him, but Gerasim's strength and vitality did not mortify but soothed him.'
>
> (Tolstoy, 1960; p. 137)

Tolstoy observed that not all people who even want to, are capable of successfully caring for another. Not all nurses, for example, manage to commit themselves adequately to the welfare of their patients. This insight is currently the topic of much debate among nurse theorists. Ivan Ilych's wife really wanted to 'nurse' him. She wanted to care for her husband. Her well-intentioned but misguided deceit provoked distrust in Ivan Ilych who preferred quiet, gentle Gerasim. The commitment of Gerasim to Ivan Ilych above and beyond what could be considered the call of duty, is illuminating. As the patient awakens at three in the morning, stiff, in pain, with the candles still lit, he is made aware of the presence of Gerasim who was:

> ' . . . sitting at the foot of the bed dozing quietly and patiently, while he himself lay with his emaciated stockinged legs resting on Gerasim's shoulders . . . "Go away, Gerasim", he whispered. "It's all right, sir. I'll stay a while." "No, go away."'
>
> (Tolstoy, 1960; p. 146)

Such scenes are repeated continuously, wherever a caring individual, professional or lay, attends to a sick or incapacitated friend, relative or patient.

As nurses we are urged to manifest a caring attitude toward our patients and caring has been postulated as the very heart of what the nursing profession is concerned with (Leininger, 1984a; Watson, 1985; Roach, 1985). Fostering a sense of commitment which is central to the concept of caring must also, therefore, be of grave concern to the profession. Commitment can be said to be a form of engagement, an undertaking or even obligation to be with a patient, not to abandon a patient – literally or figuratively. This commitment, however, like interpersonal commitments among friends or family members, does not come automatically. It is not an added, superfluous attribute of a qualified nurse. Unfortunately, there are only too many examples of nurses who have broken their pledge and therefore abandoned their commitment to patients by overtly or indirectly abusing and neglecting them.

It is not by listing horrendous tales of patient abuse, however, that lessons in the need for better nurse-patient relationships and sounder patient covenants will be achieved. Likewise, examples of non-commitment to entire peoples and sections of society are well known to us already; e.g. the abandonment of paediatric patients and AIDS patients in Romania by the erstwhile nursing and medical profession is a sad opportunistic example of lack of professional commitment to a whole group of patients. The Romanian situation is sobering also, because it highlights the possible extreme consequences of what may happen to a profession if there is insufficient commitment to nursing by its members.

Whereas in the context of discussing caring in nursing there is the temptation to simply limit oneself to an analysis of the construct of commitment as it affects the patient. It also needs to be mentioned that no commitment to a patient will last very long, or be necessarily effective, if there is no primary commitment to the profession of nursing itself. The task of fostering this type of commitment is separate from and a *sine qua non* to that of fostering an ability to achieve and maintain therapeutic relationships among patients.

The whole notion of love of one's work and commitment to its ideals is necessary for a health profession and is the subject of much intra-professional debate. Ever since Kramer (1972) announced to the stunned nursing world that the lofty ideals of nursing students can be quickly shattered and broken, and that neophyte nurses can become brutalised and embittered by the realisation that *care* is not always the driving force among working nursing professionals, the literature and research on burn-out and stress among nurses has burgeoned. Obviously more research is needed on various aspects of promoting a sense of commitment towards patients and among nurses towards their own professional aims and goals. Certainly the lack of professional commitment to the declared aims of the nursing profession can mean, in an extreme form, the very annihilation of that profession, as in the previously mentioned sad case of Romania.

Commitment in any form involves courage and fortitude, as Saint-Exupery commented on the moral greatness of his friend Guillaumet, stranded in the snow-storms of the Andes, 'His moral greatness consists in his sense of responsibility'; responsibility which propelled him onwards and forbade him to give up or to capitulate. Just as Guillaumet recognised that what saved him from freezing to death was taking one small step after another – 'What saves a man is to take a step. Then another step. It is always the same step, but you have to take it.' (Saint Exupery, 1967; p. 42). So what prevents a nurse from taking responsibility for her patient's welfare is her frequent fear of commitment which is manifested by fear of engagement. It is a sad truism, however, to say that without engagement there will not only be avoidance of painful encounters, but also of uplifting and mutually growth-inducing experiences. Guillaumet willed himself to survive because 'he knew that he was responsible for himself, for the mails, for the fulfilment of the hopes of his comrades. He was holding in his hands their sorrow and their joy . . . Responsible in as much as his work contributed to it, for the fate of those men' (Saint-Exupery, 1967); and Saint-Exupery makes no doubt about the fact that he thought Guillaumet was exceptional, brave and thoroughly committed. The modern nurse must be equally committed to the patient, her colleagues, and to at least one more concept, namely health (Van Hooft, 1987).

Van Hooft, in a fascinating and thought-provoking article on commitment to health as an achievable nursing goal, comments on the heady idealism that modern nurse-theorists imply in their caring theories. He notes that caring theories call for a particular moral orientation on the part of nurses (Van Hooft, 1987) and yet this can produce lowered work morale in the long-term, because it simply is not always possible to be adequately committed to all patients.

> ' . . . and this is not just because there will not be time enough; it's just not going to be psychologically possible either. A manageable professional life will need to have limited and *attainable* goals.'
> (Van Hooft, 1987; emphasis mine)

One of the main 'limited and attainable goals' of nursing is a fostered commitment to the promotion, restoration and maintenance of health and well-being. As Van Hooft wisely adds:

> 'Guidelines for this might be meaningfully sought and formulated, but at least the nurse will not be confronted with an unattainably vague requirement to become responsible for a client's *whole life*.'
> (Van Hooft, 1987; emphasis mine)

According to Van Hooft, a nurse's experience and sensitivity will guide the level of commitment to health necessary to promote the client/patient welfare, and 'the basis upon which one is able to make such judgements is training and reflection' (Van Hooft, 1987). Thus, for Van Hooft, commitment, especially the nurse's commitment to the promotion of health is understood as an 'existential stance' (Van Hooft, 1987). As nurse theorists, Saint-Exupery, Tolstoy and many others have observed, commitment involves the giving of self at the deepest of levels, it

> ' . . . implicates one's deepest self. It does this because it arises from one's deepest self and goes on to constitute that self. All one's hopes, loves, fears, character traits, habits and skills come to expression in the commitments that one makes.'
>
> (Van Hooft, 1987)

Commitment to health, to its promotion, restoration and maintenance, together with a commitment to the patient as a person with whom we have the conscious courage to express solidarity, as well as commitment to the profession of nursing as a vehicle for the attainment of the former, carries with it a certain degree of heightened expectation. It is Van Hooft who aptly notes that:

> 'insofar as a commitment may be public, it sets up expectations which others then have the right to impose upon us;'

often thereby forcing us to alter our hitherto held convictions or stance. We reorganise our priorities and become prepared to sacrifice ourselves for our new found values. Thus 'the nurse will feel that certain sorts of assistance "must" be rendered; that it would be a failure of commitment not to do so' (Van Hooft, 1987).

According to Van Hooft (1987), the object of commitment is health 'as an ideal to be realised in persons, and the attitude that should grow from this is a concern for such health'. Van Hooft's theory of health commitment has much to offer in the construction of the caring paradigm. He argues eloquently that it is the health of a person that is the object of a nurse's concern more than the person as such which, although a contestable notion by many caring theorists, is certainly a notion worthy of examination. Undoubtedly, concern about health issues, commitment to restoration of a patient's health, and care to maintain a person's health, are all endeavours inherent in the nurse's avowed intent of 'caring for patients'. Finally, it is Van Hooft's proposition that

> 'the therapeutically required rapport between nurse and client will have to be established on the basis of their mutual perception of

the nurse's professional commitment to caring for health. This caring, even though it is not for the whole person, should be sufficient to establish the trust in the nurse that the patient needs to feel.'

(Van Hooft, 1987)

If, according to Roach (1985), commitment is a 'complex affective response characterised by a convergence between one's desires and one's obligations, and by a deliberate choice to act in accordance with them', it should not surprise us that to be professionally committed requires considerable forethought and courage and even political and legal awareness. Sometimes this is manifested by standing up for patients' rights, and by being a patient's advocate, especially when professional insight dictates the presence of potential abuse.

In conclusion, Roach's five behavioural elements of caring; compassion, competence, confidence, conscience and commitment although discreet entities, can be seen to overlap and at times to merge. The caring phenomena inevitably, is a far greater and awesome occurance than any intellectual summation of its constituent parts. For purposes of professional progress however, such an analytical approach is essential. The most important and significant aspect of caring, however, is that delicate re-integration and synthesis of knowledge, skills, commitment, professional integrity and love manifested each time a professional nurse consciously undertakes to nurse a patient or client. This is done because the nurse cares.

References

Akinsanya, J. (1986). A professional knowledge base. *Senior Nurse*, **4(3)**, 6–8.

Barber, P. (1991). Caring – the nature of a therapeutic relationship. In *Nursing: A Knowledge Base For Practice*. A. Perry and M. Jolley (Eds), pp. 230–70. Edward Arnold, London.

Beauvoir, S. de (1973). *A Very Easy Death*. Warner, New York.

Benner, P. (1984). *From Novice to Expert*. Addison–Wesley, Menlo Park.

Benner, P. and Wrubel, J. (1989). *The Primacy Of Caring*. Addison–Wesley, Menlo Park.

Bergman, R. (1981). Accountability – definition and dimensions. *International Nursing Review*, **28(2)**, 53–9.

Boykin, A. and Schoenhofer, S. (1990). Caring in nursing: analysis of extant theory. *Nursing Science Quarterly*, **3(4)**, 149–55.

Brown L. (1986). The experience of care: patient perspectives. *Topics in Clinical Nursing*, **8(2)**, 56–62.

Burnard, P. (1988). Empathy: the key to understanding. *Professional Nurse*, **3(10)**, 388–91.

Campbell, A. V. (1984). *Moderated Love: A Theology Of Professional Care*. SPCK, London.

Campbell, A. V. (1985). *Paid to Care? The Limits Of Professionalism In Pastoral Care*. SPCK, London.

Campbell, A. V. (1988). Profession and vocation. In: *Ethical Issues In Caring*. G. Fairbairn and S. Fairbairn (Eds), pp. 1–9, Avebury, Aldershot.

Carper, B. A. (1979). The ethics of caring. *Advances in Nursing Science*, **1(3)**, 11–9.

Cooper M. C. (1990). Chronic illness and nursing's ethical challenge. *Holistic Nursing Practice*, **5(1)**, 10–6.

Cronin, S. N. and Harrison, B. (1988). Importance of nursing caring behaviours as perceived by patients after myocardial infarction. *Heart and Lung*, **17(4)**, 374–80.

Darbyshire, P. (1990). The heart of the matter. *Nursing Times*, **86(47)**, 63–4.

Darbyshire, P. (1991). The American revolution. *Nursing Times*, **87(6)**, 57–8.

Dunlop, M. J. (1986). Is a science of caring possible? *Journal of Advanced Nursing*, **11(6)**, 661–70.

Erikson, E. H. (1963). Childhood and Society. 2nd edn. Norton, New York.

Forrest, D. (1989). The experience of caring. *Journal of Advanced Nursing*, **14(10)**, 815–23.

Forsyth, D., Delaney, C., Maloney, N., Kubesh, D. and Story D. (1989). Can caring behavior be taught? *Nursing Outlook*, **37(4)**, 164–6.

Fry, S. T. (1988). The ethic of caring: can it survive in nursing? *Nursing Outlook*, **36(1)**, 48.

Fry, S. T. (1989). Toward a theory of nursing ethics. *Advances in Nursing Science*, **11(4)**, 9–22.

Gaut, D. A. (1981). Conceptual analysis of caring: research method. In: *Caring: An Essential Human Need. Proceedings of Three National Caring Conferences*. M. Leininger (Ed), pp. 17–24. Slack, Thorofare.

Gaut, D. A. (1983). Development of a theoretically adequate description of caring. *Western Journal of Nursing Research*, **5(4)**, 313–24.

Gaut, D. (1984). A theoretic description of caring as action. In *Care: the Essence Of Nursing and Health*. M. Leininger (Ed), pp. 27–44. Slack, Thorofare.

Gaut, D. A. (1986). Evaluating caring competencies in nursing practice. *Topics in Clinical Nursing*, **8(2)**, 77–83.

Gaylin, W. (1976). *Caring*. Knopf, New York.

Gaylin, W. (1985). Feelings. In *Powers That Make Us Human: the*

Foundation Of Medical Ethics. K. Vaux (Ed), pp. 55–73. University of Illinois Press, Urbana.

Geissler, E. M. (1990). An exploratory study of selected female registered nurses: meaning and expression of nurturance. *Journal of Advanced Nursing*, **15(5)**, 525–30.

Gilligan, C. (1982). *In a Different Voice*. Harvard University Press, Cambridge.

Gould, D. (1990). Empathy: a review of the literature with suggestions for an alternative research strategy. *Journal of Advanced Nursing*, **15(10)**, 1167–74.

Griffin, A. P. (1983). A philosophical analysis of caring in nursing. *Journal of Advanced Nursing*, **8(4)**, 289–95.

Hall, B. A. (1990). The struggle of the diagnosed terminally ill person to maintain hope. *Nursing Science Quarterly*, **3(4)**, 177–84.

Hamilton, E. and Cairns, H. (Eds), (1961). *The Collected Dialogues Of Plato*. Princeton University Press, Princeton. (Bollingen Series 71).

Hare, R. M. (1981). *Moral Thinking: Its Levels, Method and Point*. Oxford University Press, Oxford.

Hauerwas, S. (1985). Virtue. In *Powers That Make Us Human: the Foundation Of Medical Ethics*. K. Vaux (Ed), pp. 117–40. University of Illinois Press, Urbana.

Henderson, V. (1978). The concept of nursing. *Journal of Advanced Nursing*, **3(2)**, 113–30.

Henderson, V. A. (1980). Preserving the essence of nursing in a technological age. *Journal of Advanced Nursing*, **5(3)**, 245–60.

Holden, R. J. (1990). Empathy: the art of emotional knowing in holistic nursing care. *Holistic Nursing Practice*, **5(1)**, 70–9.

Hutchinson, S. A. (1990). Responsible subversion: a study of role bending among nurses. *Scholary Inquiry for Nursing Practice*, **4(1)**, 3–17.

Jolley, M. (1989). The professionalization of nursing: the uncertain path. In *Current Issues In Nursing*. M. Jolley and P. Allan (Eds), pp. 1–22. Chapman and Hall, London.

Kitson, A. (1985). On the concept of nursing care. In: *Ethical Issues In Caring*, G. Fairbairn and S. Fairbairn (Eds), pp. 21–31. Avebury, Aldershot.

Kohlberg, L. (1986). Moral stages and moralization: the cognitive-developmental approach. In *Moral Development and Behavior Theory: Research and Social Issues*. T. Lickona (Ed), pp. 31–5. Holt Rinehart and Winston, New York.

Kramer, M. (1974). *Reality Shock: Why Nurses Leave Nursing*. Mosby, St Louis.

Labelle, H. (1978). Nursing authority. *Journal of Advanced Nursing*, **3(2)**, 145–154.

Lanara, V. A. (1982). Responsibility in nursing. *International Nursing Review*, **29(1)**; 7–10.

Leininger, M. M. (1978). *Transcultural Nursing: Concepts, Theories and Practice*. Wiley, New York.

Leinginer, M. M. (1981). Cross cultural hypothetical functions of caring and nursing care. In *Caring: An Essential Human Need. Proceedings of Three National Caring Conferences*. M. Leininger (Ed), pp. 96–102. Slack, Thorofare.

Leininger, M. (1984a). Care: the essence of nursing and health. In *Care: the Essence Of Nursing and Health*. M. M. Leininger (Ed). pp. 3–15. Slack, Thorofare.

Leininger, M. M. (Ed), (1984b). *Care: The Essence Of Nursing and Health*. Slack, Thorofare.

Leininger, M. M. (1986). Care facilitation and resistance factors in the culture of nursing. *Topics in Clinical Nursing*, **8(2)**, 1–12.

Leininger, M. and Watson, J. (Eds), (1990). *The Caring Imperative In Education*. National League for Nursing, New York.

Levine, M. (1977). Nursing ethics and the ethical nurse. *American Journal of Nursing*, **77(5)**, 845–9.

Liehr, P. R. (1989). The core of true presence: a loving center. *Nursing Science Quarterly*, **2(1)**, 7–8.

Manley, K. (1991). Knowledge for nursing practice. In *Nursing: A Knowledge Base For Practice*. A. Perry and M. Jolley (Eds), pp. 1–27. Edward Arnold, London.

Maslow, A. H. (1970). *Motivation and Personality*. 2nd edn. Harper and Row, New York.

Mayer, D. K. (1986). Cancer patients' and families' perception of nurse caring behaviours. *Topics in Clinical Nursing*, **8(2)**, 63–9.

Mayeroff, M. (1971). *On Caring*. Harper and Row, New York.

McFarlane, J. (1988). Nursing: a paradigm of caring. In *Ethical Issues In Caring*. G. Fairbairn and S. Fairbairn (Eds), pp. 10–20. Avebury, Aldershot.

Meerabeau, L. (1991). The presentation of competence in health care. *Journal of Advanced Nursing*, **16(1)**, 63–7.

Meize-Grochowski, M. (1984). An analysis of the concept of trust. *Journal of Advanced Nursing*, **9(6)**, 563–72.

Moccia, P. (1988). At the faultline: social activism and caring. *Nursing Outlook*, **36(1)**, 30–3.

Morrison, P. (1989). Nursing and caring: a personal construct theory study of some nurses' self-perceptions. *Journal of Advanced Nursing*, **14(5)**, 421–6.

Morse, J. M., Solberg, S. M., Neander, W. L., Bottorff, J. L. and Johnson, J. L. (1990). Concepts of caring and caring as a concept. *Advances in Nursing Science*, **13(1)**, 1–14.

Murdoch, I. (1970). *The Sovereignty Of Good*. Routledge and Kegan Paul, London.

Noddings, N. (1984). *Caring: A Feminine Approach to Ethics and Moral Education*. University of California Press, Berkeley.

Orlando, I. J. (1961). *The Dynamic Nurse-Patient Relationship*. Putnam, New York.

Parse, R. R. (1981). Caring from a human science perspective. In *Caring An Essential Human Need. Proceedings of Three National Caring Conferences*. M. Leininger (Ed), pp. 129–32. Slack, Thorofare.

Pepper, C. B. (1985). The roles of care and love and hope between nurse and patient in cancer survival. *Cancer Nursing*, **8**, Supplement 1; 50–3.

Piaget, J. (1932). *Moral Judgement Of the Child*. Routledge & Kegan Paul, London.

Powell, J. H. (1989). The reflective practitioner in nursing. *Journal of Advanced Nursing*, **14(10)**, 824–32.

Rawnsley, M. M. (1985). Nursing: the compassionate science. *Cancer Nursing*, **8**, (Suppl. 1), 71–4.

Rawnsley, M. (1990). Of human bonding: the context of nursing as caring. *Advances in Nursing Science*, **13(1)**, 41–8.

Ray, M. A. (1981). A philosophical analysis of caring within nursing. In *Caring: An Essential Human Need. Proceedings of Three National Caring Conferences*. M. Leininger (Ed), pp. 25–36. Slack, Thorofare.

Raya, A. (1990). Can knowledge be promoted and values ignored? Implications for nursing education. *Journal of Advanced Nursing*, **15(5)**, 504–9.

Roach, S. M. (1985). A foundation for nursing ethics. In *Nursing Law and Ethics*. A. Carmi and S. Schneider (Eds), pp. 170–7. Springer-Verlag, Berlin.

Saint-Exupery, A. de (1967). *Wind, Sand and Stars*. Harcourt Brace Jovanovich, New York.

Saint-Exupery, A. de (1989). *Southern Mail*. Penguin, London.

Samarel, N. (1990). Said another way: please don't leave me alone. *Nursing Forum*, **25(2)**, 31–4.

Scudder, J. R. (1990). Dependent and authentic care: implications of Heidegger for nursing care. In *The Caring Imperative In Education*. M. Leininger and J. Watson (Eds), pp. 59–66. National League for Nursing.

Smith, M. J. (1990). Caring: ubiquitous or unique. *Nursing Science Quarterly*, **3(2)**, 54.

Smith, P. (1991). The nursing process: raising the profile of emotional care in nursing training. *Journal of Advanced Nursing*, **16(1)**, 74–81.

Solzenitsyn, A. (1969). *Cancer Ward*. Bantam Books, New York.

Toliver, J. C. (1988). Inductive reasoning: critical thinking skills for clinical competence. *Clinical Nurse Specialist*, **2(4)**, 174–9.

Tolstoy, L. (1960). *The Death Of Ivan Ilych and Other Stories*. Signet, New York.

Van Hooft, S. (1987). Caring and professional commitment. *Australian Journal of Advanced Nursing*, **4(4)**, 29–38.

Van Hooft, S. (1990). Moral education for nursing decisions. *Journal of Advanced Nursing*, **15(2)**, 210–5.

Van Langingham, J. (1984). Guilt. In *Introduction To Nursing: An Adaptation Model*. 2nd edn. C. Roy (Ed), pp. 376–93. Prentice-Hall, Englewood Cliffs.

Watson, J. (1981). Some issues related to a science of caring for nursing practice. In *Caring: An Essential Human Need. Proceedings of Three National Caring Conferences*. M. Leininger (Ed), pp. 61–8. Slack, Thorofare.

Watson, J. (1985). *Nursing: the Philosophy and Science Of Caring*. Colorado Associated University Press, Boulder.

Watson, M. J. (1988). New dimensions of human caring theory. *Nursing Science Quarterly*, **1(4)**, 175–81.

Watson, J. (1990). Caring knowledge and informed moral passion. *Advances in Nursing Science*, **13(1)**, 15–24.

Wolf, Z. R. (1986). The caring concept and nurse identified caring behaviors. *Topics in Clinical Nursing*, **8(2)**, 84–93.

2 Values and philosophy in nursing: the dynamic of change?

In 1977 at an interview for nurse training I was asked politely but cynically what theology and philosophy (my degree subjects) had to do with nursing. My answer was that they were the theoretical side of the practical nursing coin. They were to do with life and death questions, understanding humanity and the value that we give to ourselves. Thirteen years later the very values in question have become fashionable. They are seen to be of worth, hence the inclusion of this chapter in a publication on current nursing issues. A change in ideas appears to have brought with it a change in values, but in fact the converse has happened. A change in values has brought about new ideas. In the first half of this chapter I shall attempt to look at the nature of these values, old and new, and discuss their implications for nursing practice. In the second part I shall look at the place of philosophy in nursing and in the third part offer some suggestions of my own.

Part 1

Nursing values

'Becoming a nurse is not simply a matter of learning particular skills, in adopting forms of behaviour appropriate to a particular context. It is also a matter of coming to know the values of a profession in a way which can profoundly influence the thinking, personality and lifestyle of the individual concerned.'

(Thompson *et. al.*, 1983)

These contemporary words are undoubtedly true of any employment past or present which in former days would have called itself a vocation. Thirty years ago no one would have doubted that nursing was a vocation. It was very soundly rooted in a Christian ethos, both historically and culturally. A sense of duty, a slightly suspicious phrase nowadays, refashioned as accountability, was considered of supreme value:

46

'Nurses very much need a strong sense of duty to enable them to care for irritating and ungrateful people, when their bodies are crying out for rest and their minds for peace. And there are years and years of it ahead. People are seldom at their best when they are sick.'

(Way, 1962)

This realistic description would not grace a current Department of Health recruitment advertisement, but it does begin to paint a picture of the nurse of the time. Other valuable qualities were 'self control, assurance, observation, punctuality, cleanliness, truthfulness, confidence, anticipation and firmness', (Way, 1962). Unquestionably nurse 1950s was nice and good. Way goes on to state that:

'Matters of moral value fade imperceptibly into matters of etiquette. The unwritten laws of nursing spring largely from the religious and moral character of most of its pioneers.'

(Way, 1962).

The other virtue of nurses which was supremely valuable to nursing itself and to medicine more particularly was that they did as they were bid and knew their place:

'Ward routine has a certain pattern to encourage respect for the doctor. He is always accompanied by the Sister, the ward is quiet, he is never contradicted, and by various means he is shown to be a person of pre-eminent skill and wisdom.'

(Way, 1962).

The implications for nursing of the values held by most nurses and more importantly by society in general, are retrospectively obvious. Nursing was an orderly affair based on the medical model. It borrowed its academic body of knowledge from medicine and developed its practical skills around that knowledge. Not that we should underestimate those skills which were considerable and passed down from Sister to staff in a fashion akin to the oral tradition. Work was necessarily task-orientated because of the authoritarian values of the time.

'Authority means security. It is necessary to realise that the actions of authority really spring from love.'

(Way, 1962).

The virtues valued in a good nurse were necessarily not characteristics which could be switched off when she was not at work. There was no division between behaviour in professional and personal life as the boarding school regulations of nurses' homes testified. One was never really 'off duty'. These nurses were not, of course, the novice-like creatures they were supposed to be. How desperately boring nursing would have been if they had been. My mother, I am sure, was not alone in dodging the Home Sister and climbing in through the window after curfew hours following some totally innocent but exciting escapade. Nonetheless a strict moral code was upheld both overtly, (many voluntary hospitals pre 1948 were run by nuns and many subsequent NHS hospitals held ward prayers in the morning) and subliminally (morals and etiquette merged) and it was Victorian–Christian in character. That is to say it was soundly rooted in the Christian principles of service – healing and love of mankind, but could not avoid a cultural milieu which was still smarting from strict codes of Victorian manners.

Ten years ago I would have bristled at the above images of male medical dominance over humble, if not humiliated, nursing. Now it seems so ridiculous as to be funny. Why was it that humility was a prized value 30 years ago, a bone of contention 15 years ago and virtually forgotten now with the acquisition of assertiveness? The answer would appear to be that values have changed. This is, of course, not at all extraordinary. British society has altered enormously in the last 30 years and nursing would have been an anachronism if it had not done so too. The way that society views and values nurses has also altered in this period. The 'man in the street' would now, as 30 years ago, say that nurses are 'marvellous'. However before the Second World War nurses in a violent and vicious East End of London did not fear for personal safety. Everywhere now nurses are the subject of violent physical and sexual attacks. Page 3 tabloid double 'd' cup nursing fantasies show the real value placed on nursing by many in contemporary masculine society.

To describe the causes of change in society and hence in nursing over the last 30 years would be an historical and sociological exercise which is not the remit of this chapter, but I would wish to draw attention to what I believe to be major factors in nursing change, e.g. the rise of the women's movement; a period of liberal politics followed by a new conservatism; technological and scientific advances; and a change from a society which was predominantly, even if nominally, Christian to a pluralistic one which has precipitated an anarchy of belief and value in certain spheres of life. I shall make some references to these projected causes whilst discussing the major areas of nursing in which an alteration in values has appeared most prominently. These would include the following:

- The drive for professionalism
- The establishment of nursing theory, nursing models and the nursing process
- The nursing curriculum
- The image of the nurse

The drive for professionalism

The attainment of professional status would be seen by many nurses as the zenith of nursing history; the achievement of just recognition for what they value in nursing, its dedication, strength, service, skill and usefulness. The feelings of equality and independence nurtured by the women's movement and a time of cultural liberalism in the 1960s and 1970s became in a more conservative 1980s, a rebellious conformity; the desire to compete with others. Professional status would put nursing on a near equal, if not totally equal, footing with medicine (the value of power) and strengthen not only nurses themselves but their role as patient advocates. The struggle has not however been viewed uncritically by all nurse observers. As Schröck comments:

'The generally ready acceptance by nurses of the functionalist approach to professionalism is uncritical, superficial and ineffective. . . . just to fulfil the traditional criteria of the profession is going to lead no further than mystification of the public and self deception.'

(Schröck, 1987)

Ruth Schröck does nonetheless feel that a critical examination and re-thinking of the professional role can lead to nurses sharing in power rather than being controlled by circumstances:

'It creates the potential for nurses as an occupational group to contribute to constructive social change, towards a more open professionalism and a more open and, therefore, humane and compassionate society.'

(Schröck, 1987)

The problem with these generally wise and appealing words is that Dr Shröck wishes to 'have it both ways'. Professionalism is by definition a closed affair and cannot be made open to match one's ideals. The values which are being striven for are twofold. There is a desire, as there has ever been, to do good – to serve; that is to bring about effective social change, alongside the desire (need) for the power to do these things and the respect befitting one with such power. There is an element of self value in the search for professionalism which is strident and in itself powerful. It is this which has intimidated many of medicine's onlookers. The radical nursing critics of professionalism such as Jane Salvage are condemnatory not of the development of self value and self determination but of what they see as its misguided vehicle. She comments that:

'The political demands of professionalism for better pay, more status and so on – are inseparable from its effects on nursing work. The attempt to win recognition and attendant material benefits for a selected group inevitably exclude others, and insisting on strict control of entry and education, and therefore knowledge, denies it to others, not least the patients themselves. The rarer the commodity, the more it's worth – ask Harley Street – but do we really want nursing to travel that road?'

(Salvage, 1985)

Whether the bid for professionalism is appropriate or inappropriate what nurses are saying by it is, "We have highly developed and worthy skills, technological and scientific knowledge and we are necessary and productive. *We* are of value".

Nursing theory, nursing models and the nursing process

The evolution of the professional nurse and of nursing theory have necessarily come hand in hand. A professional needs a body of knowledge and having this knowledge means that one can begin to strive for professional status. To our mother's generation, to ask what it meant to be a 'nurse' or what it meant to 'care' would have been 'crackpot' questions. You might ask *what* a nurse did, or *how* she cared for someone, but not what its significance was. One nurse of her generation did, however, and she was Virginia Henderson whose model is the backbone of modern nursing literature. The need to analyse the structure and purpose of her work and decipher the values on which it was built were necessary to her and many years later have apparently become necessary to nursing in this country. Indeed, the most interesting aspect of the advent of nursing theory/nursing models is the statement of values that they display. For in as much as they analyse the nature of nursing itself (to steal from Henderson) they are statements of belief in the values of society and nursing's relationships to it.

The main emphasis shared by all major nursing models has been to redress the devaluation of the person which appeared to happen by seeing a purely physiological entity as in the medical model. (*See* Chapter 5). In order to do this the 'nature' of the person has to be assessed and described. Philosophically this is an extraordinary arrogance. Henderson's assessment remains more deeply profound than most of its successors, probably due to its intentional simplicity (Henderson, 1966). Having defined those areas of need and value to the person, the areas of skill and value to the nurse can then be correlated. Models aim to do more than philosophical assessment. They aim to structure a pattern for care and initiate a mode of thinking and acting in the role of the nurse. The theme of most models has been to place value upon man as a biological, psychological and sociological entity. The value is allegedly upon the 'whole' person although the language used in many models has tended to show them as somewhat mechanistic and disjointed. Aggleton and Chalmers (1986) state that:

'The Johnson Behavioural Systems Model of nursing encourages nurses to see individuals as having a set of interrelated behavioural sub-systems, each striving for balance and equilibrium within itself.'

'Roy's model of nursing argues that there exist four principle systems of adaptation influencing behaviour. These are called modes of adaptation, and they comprise the physiological, self concept, role function, and interdependency systems.'
(Aggleton and Chalmers, 1986)

Critics of the systems approach to humanity emphasize that it is a purely Western one and that a truly holistic approach would not fragment people in such a way. Martha Rogers in her holistic vision sees people as 'unitary fields of energy interacting with other energy fields in their vicinity', and the role of the nurse is described as promoting 'symphonic interaction between man and environment, to strengthen the coherence and integrity of the human field, and to direct and redirect patterning of the human and environmental fields for realisation of maximum health potential' (Aggleton and Chalmers, 1986).

The tragedy of these nursing models is that they have attempted to leave behind the purely physiological (scientific) view of man as a one-dimensional creature and have succeeded only, perhaps with the exception of Henderson, in creating nothing but *a more complicated* one-dimensional being. The language of description is scientific or indeed pseudoscientific, and even Rogers' attempts to describe a whole person are quasi scientific. Her descriptions have no rational basis. They are symbolic. The symbol is a profoundly useful tool but it needs imagery and universal accessability, not incomprehensible jargon borrowed from nouveau scientific trends.

Contemporary nurse theorists would argue that task orientation and the medical model devalued humanity by making people into 'things' to be practised upon. Nursing models, they would insist, recreate for the nurse a person with whom one can relate. They have, however, further objectified the person rendering authentic manifestation of the truth, and all descriptions must conform to its boundaries. Humanity, however, does not. Our mothers' generation knew this and that is why they did not ask 'crackpot' questions.

The nursing process (*see* Chapter 4) has not only attempted to

systematise nursing but to involve patients in the process on a partnership basis. The person is not seen as 'a disease with symptoms' but
as 'a patient with needs' (Chapman, 1985), and when the nursing
process is at its best those needs can be described by the patient
himself, not merely imputed by the carer. The nursing process is
ideally a statement of organisation and co-operative valuing the care
giver and the recipient as equal partners. Unfortunately in practice this
goal is not always realised and the 'person with needs' can be just as
devalued as the 'disease with symptoms'. Illich described this type of
'advance' as 'the age of disabling professions', an age when people had
'problems', experts had 'solutions' and scientists measured imponder-
ables such as 'abilities and needs' (Illich, 1977). For Illich and his co-
thinkers even patient participation in a professional-client relationship
is a grossly devaluing experience, because it creates 'needs' within
people which may not exist.

> 'While individualising need may disable by removing people from
> the social context, the compartmentalisation of the person re-
> moves even the potential for individual action. People are, in-
> stead, a set of pieces in need, both in time and space. Hopefully
> the pieces can be put together again to make a human unit of
> sufficient residual effectiveness to pay for "its" reservicing.'
>
> (McKnight, 1977)

McKnight cites the work of Elizabeth Kubler-Ross as the epitome of
this type of fragmentation, as seen in her description of five stages of
dying, each needing a new set of helpers.

There are, of course, many people whose dying relatives have been
cared for by the Hospice movement which has generally accepted
Kubler-Ross' interpretation of dying and who would feel an immense
gratitude to her for the way in which their loved ones were helped and
understood, albeit 'stage by stage'. The point to be learned from
radical critics such as Illich and McKnight, whose reflections pre-date
modern nursing theory, is a salient one all the same. Professional
theory in general and nursing theory in particular in this context have
been greatly influenced by the prevailing ethos of the time which is a
western, materialist, rationalist, scientific and pseudoscientific, objec-
tifying view of the world. The danger for the person valuing these
ideals is that the person himself may become devalued.

The nursing curriculum

The above description of an objective philosophy underlying nursing
values appears to leave one glaring omission. No explanation is left
either for motivation or for the compassionate altruistic sentiments

still experienced in nursing. It is clear that a Christian value system no longer operates overtly, although there are still many practising Christians in nursing and it is difficult to assess what subliminal influence hundreds of years of Christian morality still has upon contemporary society. Most nurses are not Christians, a few will belong to other major religions and some will be either atheistic or agnostic. For the vast majority, however, religion will be utterly meaningless. I draw a contrast between this state and the atheist or the agnostic, both of whom have contemplated their position and have either positively rejected the notion of God or admitted ignorance. Both of these exercises have been purposeful. Religious matters do not form part of the mental set of most people in a secular materialist society. This is not to say, however, that the non-religious are without compassion and caring. The beliefs underpinning most contemporary nursing curricula are secular but display considerable concern for the nature of humanity. In the list below I have summarised the beliefs of a dozen nursing curricula throughout Britain. Some of these statements were incorporated in the curriculum 'philosophy'; however at this juncture I would prefer to refer to them as a list of beliefs.

- People are individuals with a right to determine their own destiny
- People are bio, psycho, social (and spiritual in some cases) entities
- People should be viewed holistically and within their cultural milieu
- Health care should be an oscillating partnership between carer and client. The former bearing more of the burden until the carer recovers enough to take responsibility for their own wellbeing
- Nurses have needs, beliefs and values of their own which need to be recognised. They also have professional responsibilities
- Education is an ongoing undertaking and students have both responsibilities and rights with respect to them
- Nurse–patient relationships should exist in an open and honest form
- Nurse management and education should be democratic, person centred and self evaluative

Two of the curricula actually use the words 'humanistic values' and it is quite clear that a discussion of humanism is necessary as a basis for the views expressed above. Humanism has been the personalising force of modern nursing theory. Its success along with that of other philosophical influences will be discussed in Part 2.

The image of the nurse

> 'You don't have to be a good scholar to be a good nurse. You just have to be intelligent, industrious, compassionate and tough.'
>
> (Gould, 1988)

This recent description of the modern nurse by a journalist/doctor is not ridiculous, or unrepresentative or very different from the image of 40 years ago. It does, however, leave out words like obedient, modest and virtuous which would have been implied if not written then. The nurse's image of herself also appears to have changed. This graduate nurse has no doubt about the value of assertiveness and self-respect:

> 'You often hear the complaint that nurses are treated as doctor's handmaidens, but when it happens it is because a nurse had allowed herself to be treated like that. I think a lot of the blame lies at our door, because we *are* clinical practitioners, we are professionals in our own right. Our training is different but it is not any less than the doctors.'
>
> (Gould, 1988).

When a candidate at interview is asked why she chose nursing the correct answer is no longer, 'I want to help people'. If that is what she actually feels it would be more prudent to talk about social obligation, nursing being a profession which involves relating to others, career mobility, academic and emotional gratification. The modern nurse must know where she is going and why, and be able to talk about it in an objective fashion. The value upon care remains high but care is no longer 'tender' and 'loving', it is a specifiable commodity for which there are corollarative qualities which have taken over from niceness and goodness. A nurse no longer has a vocation; she has a profession. She is no longer dedicated; she is professional. She is no longer moral; she is accountable. Skills have taken over from values and virtues enabling the nurse to step 'in' and 'out' of her role. She is, in a way, divorced from her own humanity. Whether the public image of the nurse has kept pace with these trends however, is debatable. An Army Major organising the Grand Parade to celebrate the Queen Mother's 90th birthday described the procession as containing 'civilians' as well as soldiers. He gave four examples of the 'civilians', 'Aberdeen Angus, nurses, dogs and racehorses.' (Today News Programme, 1991). Whether we are valued more than racehorses and less than prize bulls or vice versa is difficult to assess.

Conclusion

Bevis (1982) suggested that four major philosophical trends succeeded each other during nursing history:

- Ascestism; highly religious, devotional, self sacrificing approach
- Romanticism; emotional, idealistic, loyal to superiors and doctors – the handmaiden generation
- Pragmatism; emphasis on the practical use of objects and people. Importance of consequences of one's actions emphasised. Patients known by diagnosis and bed numbers
- Humanism; concern for the whole person, in the context of his family and society. The human being becomes central to nursing practice

Since the 1980s elementary existential principles have become affiliated to the basic humanism to give patients freedom of choice in health care.

Bevis' analysis is neat and alluring as it certainly displays major values which have influenced nursing historically and as Clay (1987) suggests, are all currently present in nursing. There is a danger, however, in viewing an analysis like this too simply. Essentially it can make the values and beliefs of an older generation of nurses appear ridiculous. This is to take correct analysis and the nurses themselves out of context. It is tempting to view current development as necessarily correct. An image of contemporary nursing is one which shouts from the rooftops its concern for the person, and displays this concern in the way that it is nominally organised, that is in a person-centred way, with respect to both patients and staff. Nurses themselves and many more patient victims of modern nursing theory may not feel so enthusiastic about its success. Conversely there is no doubt that a nurse during the London blitz, by necessity, had to consider bed numbers and diagnosis primarily; it was crisis management. To suggest that these nurses forgot the humanity of their patients would not only be a gross generalisation but also a grievous slander. The fact that they did not make a theory out of the person may have been quite simply because it was so elemental and obvious to them that it did not need mentioning. It is obvious that values inspire and indeed necessitate change, a change which is not clear-cut, and the boundaries of which are blurred because the values and mores of society alter in a patchy and straggling fashion. Values themselves however are only representatives of larger systems of ideas which may be called philosophies or ideologies and it is these that will be discussed in Part 2.

Part 2

Philosophy in nursing

An implied criticism has already been made of the practice of calling a list of statements of belief a philosophy. This is not intended as a criticism of curricula which use the phrase in such a way but of the very common misusage of the word philosophy for a group of ideas. One often hears of X's personal philosophy. It may be that X has devised a rigorous, rational, logically thought out system of ideas which may correctly be called a philosophy but it is more likely that X believes in various ideas, many of which cohere and which may be summarised by one or two larger principles. I would beg to suggest that the word philosophy should not be used here. 'Ideology' would be a better word although I see nothing more preferable than stating that X 'believes' for that is the most accurate, and indeed a highly laudable, description of the situation. There is nonetheless, such a thing as 'nursing philosophy' which refers to the notions of man, society, health, care, and so on, which I would again wish to refer to as nursing beliefs or occasionally nursing ideology. Some of the values implicit in these beliefs have been discussed in Part 1. The appropriate place for the word philosophy as yet exists in only two realms in nursing – in the description of any philosophical systems which might have influenced nursing beliefs; and in the realm of moral philosophy (ethics) which is at last becoming a significant factor in nurse education.

Have philosophical systems influenced nursing belief?

The term 'humanistic' has been used already and needs some explanation. Humanism is not a clear cut philosophy as such but a description of a belief which has been emerging since the Enlightenment and has been both the subject and implication of successive philosophies since then. (O'Connor, 1985). Coleridge used the phrase to deny the divinity of Christ (Shorter Oxford English Dictionary, 1978), but it has been more generally seen as, 'any system which puts human interests in the mind of man paramount, rejecting the supernatural; belief in God etc' (Chambers Concise Dictionary, 1985).

In nursing literature 'humanistic' and 'humanitarian' values are often seen as interchangeable, 'humanitarian' implying a concern for human affairs usually over and above systems, technology and other dehumanising obstacles as opposed to the divine realm. Joseph (1985) suggests that there are six basic tenets of humanism which are belief in:

(*i*)   Naturalism; a belief in the reality only of what can be perceived by the senses and objectively found in nature.

(*ii*)   The insistence on the unity of body and soul and emphasis on the here and now. Rejection or professed ignorance of the hereafter.

(*iii*) The search for truth by scientific method.

(*iv*)   Self determination of the human being and the right to freedom of choice.

(*v*)   The necessity of a moral system which addresses 'freedom, happiness and the progress of all mankind'.

(*vi*)   The attainment of the 'good life' (i.e. maximum potential) for all individuals.

Joseph points out that these tenets are manifest in nursing in its secular relativism; concentration on care of the person in their present situation; belief in the necessity of a scientific knowledge base; the emphasis on client choice and accountability; a commitment to the egalitarian nature of nursing care and the desire for personal growth of both client and colleague. It is certainly the case that the list of beliefs of representative nursing curricula in Part 1 coincides with Joseph's assessment.

Undoubtedly one of the largest influences in nursing has been from humanistic psychology; Abraham Maslow and Carl Rogers being the most popular exponents of this theory. It rebelled against the behaviourist and determinist supposition of earlier psychologies and thus was useful to nursing which was also rebelling against what it saw as the inhumanity of the medical model. Humanistic psychology appears to offer the best of all worlds because it comes in the guise of a scientific theory which underpins humanistic beliefs in the nature of man. Maslow's (1970) famous notion of self actualisation has had a profound influence on nursing concepts of human potential. Humanistic psychology does not pretend to be a philosophy but it is sometimes used as one and its influence has had enormous philosophical implications, as its theory has been used as the knowledge base for building systems of thought which believe themselves to be philosophies. Its criticisms come from opposite directions. Primarily it fails because it is impossible to evaluate scientifically.

> 'With its emphasis on developing one's potential, humanistic psychology has been closely associated with encounter groups and various types of "consciousness-expanding" and mystical experiences. It is more aligned with literature and the humanities than it is with science.'
>
> (Atkinson *et. al.*, 1983)

'We can no more afford to have a psychology that is humanistic at the expense of being scientific than we can afford one that is scientific at the expense of human relevance.'

(Smith, 1973, cited by Atkinson *et. al.*, 1983)

The attraction of humanistic psychology is obvious. Unfortunately the criticisms from the non-scientific world are equally valid, suggesting that humanistic psychology actually adds nothing to what has already been said by the great religions and hundreds of secular and religious writers and artists past and present. To take the above quotation one step further 'Why not use literature instead?' Humanistic psychology is American in origin and evolved alongside a much larger cultural belief pattern which in the absence of a more formal title I shall call 'West Coast Philosophy'. The hippy movement of the 1960s and 1970s in San Francisco and Los Angeles, with its non-specific emphasis on 'love', 'freedom' and 'experience yourself' had parallels in academic and formal disciplines. The cults which grew around 'gurus' like Timothy Leary and which leaned towards trends in psychoanalysis and diversions into eastern religions became more respectable and therapeutic in the late 1970s and 1980s, and have emerged in what are now considered essential core curriculum ingredients such as counselling and values clarification techniques. The emphasis is on knowing yourself and growth through the self. Their influence has been obvious in many of the value statements already described in contemporary nursing. The nickname 'West Coast Philosophy' is a slightly ironic one. It is obviously not a philosophy but a trend in ideas that happened to coincide with many others which turned away from the authority of the system, be it political, social, bureaucratic, theocratic, or scientific, and towards the autonomy and freedom of the individual, whose future lay in exploration of knowledge of the self. It is with respect to the individual and the self that we need to discuss two further areas; Eastern Philosophy and Existentialism.

The hippy movement of the 1960s also coincided with the transportation of 'Transcendental Meditation' from the east to both America and Britain. Considered slightly offbeat then, a secularised derivative, yoga, as exercise and mental relaxation, has become almost commonplace in health education. The increased popularity of holistic medicine as practised in some parts of the east has also had influence in the mainstream of care. The term 'holistic' is, if nothing else, part of everyday parlance. As with many of its influences it appears that nursing's grasp of these basic ideas has been somewhat superficial. It is very neat and easy to borrow an image such as 'holistic care' but whether it is possible to fit it into a secular western picture is another matter. The philosophies which underpin the religions of the East, particularly Buddhism, are both complex and culturally alien to us. One may be forgiven for confusing the image of the Buddhist meditating in search of satori (enlightenment) with 'being in touch with yourself on the west coast'. The goals are very different. The Buddhist is aiming to lose the individual 'self' in order to find oneness with the absolute – another name for extinction or annihilation.

> 'Just like a flame blown out by a strong wind
> "goes home" and so defies all definition,
> just so a sage from Name and Body freed,
> "goes home" and can no longer be defined.
>
> For the Extinguished One there is no measure
> and nothing is there to define him by.
> When all experiences come to an end
> the ways of language, too, have reached a stop.'
>
> (Schumann, 1973)

This is radically different from the centrality of the person which abounds in the west. I would suggest, therefore, that Eastern philosophy has actually had little if any influence on nursing practice although one or two of its central images are used and abused.

Downie and Calman (1987) in their excellent book about health care ethics briefly discuss the influence of Existentialism on some branches of psychiatry and social work, stressing the exultatory nature of the philosophy:

> 'One might say that whereas traditional academic philosophies have *discussed* the nature of human freedom the Existentialists have urged their followers to *experience* freedom and to practise it.'
>
> (Downie and Calman, 1987)

Nursing commentators are also now describing this influence with respect to the freedom of the client to choose or reject health care information. It is certainly the case in theory anyway that patient choice has increased and become recognised as a pertinent factor but I remain unconvinced regarding the influence of Existentialist theory in nursing. Downey and Calman (1987) make the point, 'It (Existentialism) stresses human freedom and choice and brings home to health workers the marked extent to which their clients lack those features, assumed to be the basic rights of man.' It is certainly true that choice is central to Existentialism but the concept must be taken in the context of the philosophy:

> 'In Satre's first novel *La Nausee*, the protagonist confronts the total meaninglessness of existence. The meaninglessness consists in the fact that things just are; they have no sufficient reason for

being as they are. They are contingent. They are absurd. If we try
to make sense out of existence we necessarily falsify it.'

(MacIntyre, 1985)

Some degree of salvation lies in the freedom to choose 'authentically';
that is, not in a pre-determined way (i.e. in bad faith). These concepts
do not fit into the somewhat optimistic view of human actualisation
and potential which nursing models describe. The Existentialistic view
of man is angst-ridden and dire and admittedly open to varying
interpretations. It has however, to be seen as a totality. The emphasis
on choice in nursing theory can and should be traced to the more
fundamental notion of the basic right of man. Freedom of choice as
Downie and Calman suggest is assumed. It is assumed in Existentialism
because it is a humanistic discipline. It is therefore also assumed in
general humanistic principles. Nursing theory shows no more than
evidence of basic humanism.

It seems that yet again an attractive convenient notion has been
stolen like a prize apple from a high and inaccessible tree. Wittgenstein
tells us that the ladder of explanation may be dispensed with once the
higher platform of understanding has been reached. He meant
however that the ladder had to be *climbed*, not used as a blunt
instrument with which to knock the prize to the ground. It would seem
therefore that the only legitimate philosophical influence which we
have traced so far in nursing is that of humanism. The development of
humanistic ideas have evolved from so many paths and over so many
centuries that it is impossible to claim any direct influence on a modern
institution. Nursing reflects the ideologies of the western, middle class
liberals, who write its scripts. These views are a combination of a
society's struggle to give a place of autonomy and respect to each and
every individual in a secular and ideologically unstable culture.

Moral philosophy and nurse education

It is necessarily the case that philosophy has made an impact on ethics
in nursing. Ethics, that is the analytical discussion of morals, is
generally a core curriculum subject and may be taught in diverse ways,
utilising value clarification; informal discussion groups; teaching of
various value systems; use of critical incidence; and in increasing
instances by use of moral philosophy. In the last five years numerous
British publications have joined the myriad American ones discussing
ethical issues. Nursing has a right to be proud of itself in the advances
that it has made in this field. There are still few medical schools which
have moral philosophy on the curriculum! However, the solution as to
how best to teach ethics to nurses is not as clear-cut as it might seem.
Ethics means moral philosophy and it would be unthinkable to a

philosopher that the subject should not be the core of an ethics course. The distinction however, between being a philosopher and being a nurse is primarily that the nurse *must* act upon her moral conclusions, the philosopher need not. Relating moral philosophy to everyday nursing is not always easy, and to try to take concepts from the one and transpose them onto the other can cause a forced unreality and render the subject meaningless to those to whom it is in fact of great importance. It would be ideal if moral philosophy were taught at school so that its principles were in some way assimilated and assumed. From thence one could launch into the practicalities of specific moral dilemmas. Many nursing students however, find moral philosophy an awesome and difficult subject. It can appear dry and over academic. At the end of an exposition of a complex but important idea one can be met with the response 'I don't agree with that'. When one asks for reasons there are none – it is simple intuitive disagreement. This too is understandable, even if infuriating. Thus, as important as moral philosophy itself is in the teaching of ethics, the teaching of the tools of philosophy, that is of rational argument, rigorous thought and critical analytical explanation is of overriding importance. This is not to say that ethical decision making should rule out emotional intuitive feelings but that philosophical rationality is the perfect tool for balancing them and putting them in perspective. If it is indeed the case that in teaching ethics nursing has incorporated the use of moral philosophy, it is also likely to be the case that the ethical decisions or stances arrived at within specific areas in nursing, will have been influenced by one or more of the following moral arguments:

> 'Caring about the welfare of a human being actually is an expression of respect for human dignity. The patient has a right to have his human needs satisfied because of his humanity. That puts the nurse under the obligation of striving to satisfy those needs.'
>
> (Raatikainen, 1989)

Ms. Raatikainen's statement is a moral one for it comments on the *obligation* of the nurse. Her use of the phrase 'respect for human dignity' is important as it is an essential theme in nursing morality. Downie and Calman (1987) have outlined a 'liberal–Kantian' view of morality as predominant in health care which combines 'elements of the moral philosophy of Kant and Mill and other liberal thinkers'. Undoubtedly, Kant's detailed views of the notion of respect for persons, of personal obligation and duty and on the intentions of the moral agent are central to nursing action. Warnock (1985) however, points out the cultural milieu from which these notions were derived and continue to exist.

'For although Kant himself insists that the moral law is "autonomous", self efficient and in particular independent of religious
belief, the moral outlook which he actually expands is clearly that
of the somewhat rigorous Christian sect in which he grew up, an
outlook which itself is sufficiently characteristic of at least Protes-
tant Christianity, and which is therefore widespread, although not
always explicit, in modern Europe.'

(Warnock, 1985)

Warnock suggests that Kant tries to create a Christian morality based,
not on the existence of God, but on the notions of the essentially
rational nature of moral obligation and man's responsibility to it. In
these terms it is difficult to assess a real Kantian influence on nursing
morality. It may be that Kant's rationality is a useful way of condoning
the subliminal Christian beliefs of society which can no longer profess a
Christian faith. Although Kant's total rejection of the existence of
moral feeling does not fit happily into much of nursing theory, it
remains the case that his principles, whether Christian by any other
name, do make an excellent starting point for a concept of health care
morality.

The influence of a Utilitarian principle of happiness (fulfilment) for
both individuals and society as a whole is certainly a traceable contemporary ethic. The NHS itself could be seen as an attempt to do 'the
greatest of good for the greatest number'. There are many well-
documented flaws in Utilitarian philosophy not least its vagueness in
the definition of 'good' or 'happiness'. However, the greatest caveat
with respect to its role in modern health care may be that further
corruption of the principle to 'the greatest good for the greatest
number at the least cost'. In the age of quality control in budget setting
one must not forget the economic philosophy of the capitalist Government which may be as forceful in shaping moral codes as any other.
It seems to be unlikely that traditional moral philosophy has greatly
influenced nursing morals, although it may do more if the subject is
taken seriously in general and nursing education, largely because
morals are shaped by beliefs. A particular philosophy may reinforce
one belief system or challenge another and indeed that is the nature
and purpose of the philosophical tool; to build up and break down in
order to see more clearly. Moral philosophy is essential to nursing, as
to every other aspect of human interest, as a working tool, but not as a
driving force for change.

Conclusion

In this section I have outlined nursing's current infatuation with
philosophy but suggested that the nature of this is superficial. Philoso-

phy, its content and perhaps more important its method, are of supreme value, but must like all other disciplines be taken in context and as a whole. Woods and Edwards (1989) put the matter most succinctly:

> 'The need for professionalism and all that entails in terms of behaviour and language may be enough to 'objectify' those in our care. Philosophy encourages us to stand back from our behaviour and from our language and address their focus, the people we care for.'
>
> (Woods and Edwards, 1989)

Philosophy does and should do just that – allow us to stand back. But as Woods and Edwards recognised, standing back is also an 'objective' experience. The motivation of modern nursing theory has been to change the objectification of the patient, but as much as sociology, psychology, and philosophy are illuminating and necessary contributions to care, they will always distance and never change the nature of a relationship – they will not bridge the gap. For Kierkegaard the only way across was a leap of faith. This will not do for a secular society, but people will still want answers to 'crackpot' questions.

Part 3

A critique of nursing values and a re-emphasis in the dynamic of change

'Does God have gums?' enquired my elder daughter when she was two years old. Neither her father the doctor, nor her mother the theologian, knew the answer so by mutual agreement we assigned the problem to the 'pending' file, noting its merit as representative of many such unanswerable questions. It was both physical and metaphysical, tangible and intangible. It touched both the world of the flesh and the world of the spirit. It was in essence 'tricky' because it concerned the fundamentals of life. It was in fact a 'crackpot' question. To assert, as I did earlier, that our mothers did not ask 'crackpot' questions was not an indictment of their lack of curiosity but an observation of their understanding of the world. For those who are secure either in their religious belief or cultural traditions, the need to question fundamental assumptions about life and meaning does not exist. If the symbols of one's culture are meaningful they do not need exploration. It is only when they no longer match the feelings they are meant to represent that analysis appears necessary. Modern nursing criticises previous notions of care as being 'merely intuitive'. It has missed the point. Care is *necessarily* intuitive, it is a feeling, which needs to be described appropriately. If the symbols of care no longer speak to us then the task in hand is not to be one of rejection but of recreation of new symbols to give meaning to change.

There will always be differences of opinion with respect to this problem. The classical, logical, positivist stance would be that all that can be described must be done so in terms of the natural world and if it cannot be so described, as Wittgenstein asserted, then better not speak of it at all. The attempts of nursing to describe care in a scientific and analytical manner are understandable. Care *must* be discussed, it *must* be criticised. However it seems that there is a confusion of terms. What must be discussed and taught and criticised are *aspects* of care, such as levels of intervention, methods of management, and criteria of judgement. 'Care' itself however, the motivation, the central core of the relationship with the patient is an emotional intuitive experience. It also has to be 'got right' but cannot be described analytically. This is where the logical positivist would stop and in a sense it is where nursing has stopped also for it has reduced the notion of care to absurdity and therefore to a standstill. To promote meaningful change one must bound from the prevalent linear model to more lateral thought. I will not call it a leap of faith (for the moment) but certainly one of the imagination. Michael Wilson, a medical doctor, priest and theologian contributes two very valuable images:

> 'If you try to convey your meaning by a series of logical arguments, it is like a chain of links. If one is broken, the sense is lost. If you can try to convey your meaning by a variety of methods – story, argument, case studies, poetry, prayer, picture or sermon – then one broken thread does not lose the meaning which is carried forward by the threads, like a rope.'
>
> (Wilson, 1988)

Nursing has placed all its value upon the objective threads and neglected the personal ones. The reader may wish to raise an objection at this point. What of the considerable emphasis and value placed upon personal skills such as communication, counselling and group dynamics? The question partly answers itself. Communication, counselling and social skills are just those. They are *skills*. They are extremely valuable and necessary to nursing and a great advancement in the care of people BUT are rendered totally meaningless outside the *relationship* of 'care'.

'In the caring professions it is possible to use ones skills as a substitute for relationship.'

(Wilson, 1988)

One of the reasons for the development of nursing devoid of the appropriate symbols may be society's own confusion over meaningful images. Contemporary cultural relativism has had the advantage of leading society away from the fundamentalist stance which historically and currently has been the cause of intolerance and persecution, not only with the popular face of Islam, but also in Christianity and Communism. The negative side of the relativist position however is the ideological anarchy which may ensue. The success of images and symbols, historically rendered through religion, would lead one to assume that imagery is important to man in order to make meaning of indescribable terms. Where there is no set doctrine, no universal symbol, man is left in a hiatus grasping for truth, for right and wrong and expression of his emotions.

'The difficulty with ethical debates is that you cannot say that one is right and the other wrong; it is often a matter of personal opinion and it is the difficulty in accepting another's views along with your own that causes the conflict.'

(Satterthwaite, 1990)

The author's statement is highly understandable but illustrates perfectly the dangerous position that relativism can lead to. It renders the science of morals a nonsense. Thompson *et. al.*, (1983) draw the following conclusion, saying that if we

'surrender our faith in reasoned argument, public debate and the possibility of social agreement then we are lost to the forces of irrationalism, prejudice and anarchy.'

This position quite rightly and necessarily removes the moral from the world of opinion to the realm of the rational but one is still left with the question 'what of faith itself'? Faith need not mean narrow-minded adherence to a particular religious tradition, but it does mean steadfast belief. We have already seen that nursing is based upon a collection of beliefs about the way the world is, about man's place in it, about the nature of care and the nature of nursing. This is faith. It need not be blind or totally irrational. It can be balanced by reason and discussion and may alter with new insights and understandings, but if it is absent then all else falls into a meaningless abyss. It might seem that relativism succeeds in allowing each to have his own faith; but to be tolerant and open to the beliefs of others is not the same as the relativist position which assumes that 'everyone can be right' for values are only

'relative to the individual'. The benefit of values clarification techniques has been to help practitioners to 'sort out their feelings' about
important issues. The danger is to take it further than it is meant to go:

> 'Values clarification incorrectly assumes that values are strictly a
> matter of individual psychology and choice. The framework pro-
> vides little opportunity for examining the quality of one's values or
> for resolving conflicts between persons who hold different values.'
> (Bernal and Bush, 1985)

Whether assumed by the theory or not it is the case that the assumption
may be made by its users. The foundation of knowing one's own
feelings which underlies counselling techniques too, has inestimable
value if not taken to be an absolute. Relativism in a sense has made the
individual absolute and rendered him devoid of 'outside help'. This
'help' need not be a belief in an objective morality but the recognition
of an external 'wisdom' to be drawn upon and to create a greater
context for one's individual feelings and values.

I have been highly critical of the advances made in nursing theory.
This is not to underestimate their enormous contribution to care if
used appropriately. The essence of the criticism is this: the dynamic of
change in nursing lies in the nature of the relationship of nurse to
patient. I reject the word client because of its economic connotations.
This relationship concerns the value placed upon one by the other and
necessitates exploration. To attempt to explore it entirely through the
sciences, social sciences or even philosophy, is like capturing a but-
terfly with a net. You have the creature but it is not really alive, nor in
its correct surroundings.

> 'They (Existentialism, Zen Buddhism and Psychoanalysis) are
> widely different in origins and general approach, but they have
> this in common that they resist the idea that the essential spirit of
> human beings can be caught in any slogan.'
> (Downie and Calman, 1987)

Existentialism and psychoanalysis are radical forms of their respective
disciplines and thus lean away from the rigidity that the sciences and
philosophy necessitate. Elsewhere Downey and Calman verge more
specifically towards the arts:

> 'The point here is that the social sciences dealing with illness must
> if they are to be sciences or respectable academic disciplines, stand
> back from the phenomenon with which they are dealing and
> present their accounts in a detached prose style of science. Litera-
> ture, on the other hand characteristically involves us directly and
> makes us physically and emotionally aware of what it is like to be

in the situation the social scientist discusses. . . . Literature has this other aspect, namely that it can sensitize sympathy or give it cognitive shaping. In other words imaginative literature can develop in a helper a perception of real need.'

(Downey and Calman, 1987)

Literature is not alone in giving us symbols for the indescribable. The famous Eduard Munch painting 'The Scream' speaks volumes about mental anguish as Verdi's *Requiem* does about grief. Moreover for the nurse/patient relationship to be a dynamic one, not only needs symbols of expression but also inspiration to see the relationship in a new light, and from ever-changing angles. One of the most dangerous and well-recognised areas of human devaluation is the objectification of the patient through pressure of work and time. An appropriate symbol can restore the true nature of relationship by lifting one out of one's linear vision. There are three symbols taken (as it happens) from religious literature which have given me a constant sense of renewal and sanity in difficult circumstances. They are: 'I and thou': 'Being there' and 'the middle way'. They are not suggested as symbols for others but examples of ways of restoring value to nursing. No matter how dedicated, moral and conscientious you are, caring for elderly people in institutional settings can be a devaluing experience for all concerned. In order *not* just to see the fifth incontinent old woman or 'another bedbath' I would try to summon up the feeling of 'I and thou' and imperceptibly the situation would change. Buber's (1958) image of contact between 'Beings' has an immediate strength which lifts those in your care from the realms of 'it'.

Being There was Peter Sellers' last film and tells the story of how a naive and simple, in the most derogatory sense of the word, gardener becomes President of the USA. The message of the film is not obvious. It is on one level a ridiculous comedy, on another, profoundly moving. A Buddhist friend of mine commented on its 'Zen nature'. The paradox of the ridiculous and the profound in some way being inextricably linked. Even its title *Being There* which has no obvious identity with the film seemed 'Zen' in its simplicity and obscurity. There are times when you don't really know what you are doing or why but there is a profound sense that you must 'be there', sharing in some perceptible way with the being of others.

'In as far as we live our lives for others, we do so not only by our actions and attitudes, but also by our interior state, what we are and what we experience most deeply inside us; the happiness and misery which come to us, the exalting and the agony we experience as individuals alone. But they are not for us alone. They are for mankind.'

(Cooper, 1974; cited by Schurr and Turner, 1982)

Margaret Cooper captures the essence of the relationship as one of shared experience, of being with another no matter how ridiculous or how profound the situation may be.

In all things one must achieve balance. It is no good holding a patient's hand and contemplating his 'thouness' if one has not tried to prevent his incontinence and remove him from an institutional form of care. But in order to see the 'person' for whom one is achieving these goals 'I and thou' may be necessary. The arts have been forgotten in the search for scientific truth; practical skills are overshadowed by academic torches. 'A middle way' is not the recipe for mediocrity but a symbol of balance and equilibrium in all things. It is a way of achieving appropriate perspectives in situations which tend to the extreme. My father-in-law when asked which pudding he would like usually makes a wise response, 'a bit of both'. The Buddha would have approved.*

These symbols are personal ones. Symbols do not need to come from religious or high-brow literature. They may be found in soap operas or cartoons or any medium which allows us to transcend ourselves in order to see another. The suggestion that the arts should play a role in nursing is not unique to this chapter. Fortunately it is being tentatively explored as an extra dimension to care. I would state the case more strongly than this. Inclusion of the arts is a medium for the understanding of values, beliefs and therefore the essence of nursing's dynamic relationship with those in its care; it is not only desirable but essential.

Conclusion

I have deliberately written this chapter in an informal style in order to emphasize the 'personal' nature of nursing which can be lost in unscientific accounts which are written in a scientific manner. In Part 1 I have attempted to show that a change in values has brought about the desire for a change in nursing theory but that the change has been a vacuous one because it has not succeeded in describing its new value system in an authentic and meaningful way. In Part 2 I have discussed the influence of philosophy in this change and suggested that its proper role is as a scientific tool of analysis but not the dynamic of change. Part 3 has been an emphatic suggestion that value and belief are at the core of nursing because of its essential *relationship* with those in care. If the nature of this relationship has changed in the last 30 years, or if it is being viewed in a different way by modern carers, then its underlying values and beliefs need to be described and explored in order for the change to be meaningful. The essential medium which is at present

---

* To assert that the picture can be made up of different aspects is *not* to say in the relativist sense that every picture is of equal value.

neglected, is the symbolic one. All changes in nursing, directly or indirectly, concerns bringing about better care. An improved understanding of 'care' would change nursing for the better. Care itself (not its aspects) cannot be analysed but it can be communicated and described in various ways given the appropriate tools. Phil Barker, a Clinical Nurse Consultant working in mental health makes the following radical and challenging statement:

> "I believe that it is incorrect to refer to any (such) interventions as 'therapy'. If nurses 'care' properly for people, then they are likely to find resolution of their life problems or else will find acceptance of their own, and others emotional, intellectual, and otherwise 'human' limitations. If nurses can find true care then there will be no need for further 'therapy'"

(Barker, 1989)

The search for true care is akin to the search for truth. Answers may be impossible but the quest is essential and will provide the dynamics of change for nursing today and tomorrow.

References

Aggleton, P. and Chalmers, H. (1986). *Nursing Models and the Nursing Process*. Macmillan, Basingstoke.

Atkinson, R. L. *et. al.* (1983). *Introduction to Psychology*. 8th edn. Harcourt Brace Jovanovich, New York.

Barker, P. (1989). Reflections on the philosophy of caring in mental health. *International Journal of Nursing Studies*. **26(2)**, 131–41.

Bernal, E. W. and Bush, E. G. (1985). Values clarification: a critique. *Journal of Nursing Education*, **24(4)**, 174–5.

Bevis, E. M. (1982). *Curriculum Building in Nursing – a Process*. 3rd edn. Mosby, St Louis.

Buber, M. (1958). *I and Thou*. T. and T. Clark, Edinburgh. *Chamber's Concise Dictionary* (1985). Chambers, Edinburgh.

Chapman, C. (1985). *Theory of Nursing: Practical Application*. Harper and Row, London.

Clay, T. (1987). *Nurses: Power and Politics*. Heinemann, London.

Downie, R. S. and Calman, K. C. (1987). *Healthy Respect: Ethics in Health Care*. Faber and Faber, London.

Gould, D. (1988). *Nurses: the Inside Story of the Nursing Profession*. Unwin Hyman, London.

Henderson, V. (1966). *The Nature of Nursing*. Macmillan, New York.

Illich, I. (1977). Disabling professions. In *Disabling Professions*, I. Illich *et. al.* (Eds), pp. 11–39. Marian Boyars, London.

Joseph, D. (1985). Humanism as a philosophy for nursing. *Nursing Forum*, **22(4)**, 135–8.

MacIntyre, A. (1985). Existentialism. In *A Critical History of Western Philosophy*, D. J. O'Connor (Ed), pp. 509–29. Macmillan, Basingstoke.

McKnight, J. (1977). Professionalized service and disabling help. In *Disabling Professions*, I. Illich *et. al.* (Eds), pp. 69–91. Marian Boyars, London.

Maslow, A. H. (1970). *Motivation and Personality*. 2nd edn. Harper and Row, New York.

O'Connor, D. J. (Ed), (1985). *A Critical History of Western Philosophy*. Macmillan, Basingstoke.

Raatikainen, R. (1989). Values and ethical principles in nursing. *Journal of Advanced Nursing*, **14(2)**, 92–6.

Salvage, J. (1985). *The Politics of Nursing*. Heinemann, London.

Satterthwaite, H. J. (1990). When right and wrong are a matter of opinion: the ethics of organ transplantation. *Professional Nurse*, **5(8)**, 434–5, 438.

Schumann, H. W. (1973). *Buddhism*. Rider, London.

Schurr, M. C. and Turner, J. (1982). *Nursing – Image or Reality*. Hodder and Stoughton, London.

Shorter Oxford English Dictionary (1978). Clarendon Press, Oxford.

Shröck, R. (1987). Professionalism – a critical examination. In *Current Issues*, L. Hockey (Ed), pp. **14** Churchill Livingstone, Edinburgh. (Recent advances in nursing 18).

Thompson, I. *et. al.* (1983). *Nursing Ethics*. Churchill Livingstone, Edinburgh.

'Today' News Programme, BBC Radio 4. 27 June 1990.

Warnock, G. J. (1985). Kant. In *A Critical History of Western Philosophy*, D. J. O'Connor (Ed), pp. 296–318. Macmillan, Basingstoke.

Way, H. (1962). *Ethics for Nurses*. Macmillan, London. (Reprinted from the *Nursing Times*).

Wilson, M. (1988). *A Coat of Many Colours*. Epworth, London.

Woods, S. and Edwards, S. (1989). Philosophy and health. *Journal of Advanced Nursing*, **14(8)**, 661–4.

3 Parsons revisited: a re-appraisal of the community nurse rôle

In this chapter some of the implications of providing care in the community will be considered. Whether the recipient is sick or healthy, to experience this care is to enter a special social world. The morality of this world reflects the morality of the prevailing social and political climate, and the rapid advancements in health care provision, along with the changed values in our society, affect the circumstances in which care is offered and the relationships between those giving and receiving care.

The World Health Organization's objective of *Health for All by the Year 2000*, has been instrumental in raising both professional and public awareness of inequalities in health. Recent legislative reforms, e.g., the National Health Service and Community Care Act 1990, and the Children Act 1989, along with the new contractual arrangement for general practitioners, are also creating new opportunities for community nurses. As a result, the demands for improved health care, offering more preventive measures and screening programmes, together with greater provision for the chronically sick, disabled and elderly, have provided incentives to change and expand services. In the community this has caused nurses to review their practice and become more involved in the promotion and facilitation of healthy life styles among client groups with whom previously they had had little contact. The care that is offered by community nurses has thus changed radically over the last decade. These trends, along with the impact of the social sciences on nurse education, have culminated in a holistic approach which seeks to respect the individuality of the patient. Each person who is approached in the home, or who presents for care in the health centre, is someone with a unique biography and personality; sickness, disease, handicap and loss affect people in different ways, and failure to differentiate between them not only does a great injustice to the singularity of the person's condition, it also fails to take account of the wider issues which constrain health choices and chances of recovery.

Since the founding of the National Health Service, the hospital sector has largely concentrated on the management and provision of care for acute illness. In addition, long-term institutional care has been provided for patients suffering from certain mental and physical

71

illnesses and handicaps, as well as for the elderly infirm. However, there has also been, especially over the last decade, a marked acceleration in the move towards caring for these patients in the community. This change in focus has provoked both problems and criticisms, and questions continue to be raised as to the appropriateness of the underlying philosophy. The dominant theme of that philosophy is the belief that by remaining in the community these client-groups will enjoy more humane treatment and a better quality of life. Sickness, both mental and physical, as well as old age, are seen as fundamental aspects of human life and experience; rather than moving people with these conditions from their homes, it is morally right and preferable for them to remain in familiar surroundings. Community care is viewed as the bridge which extends into these families and communities and which helps realize the more desirable option of having them live out their lives in their homes. Community nurses who are, in part, responsible for the interpretation and implementation of this philosophy, for redirecting care from hospitals and institutions towards the community, must be aware of the principles of benevolence and respect for patients and their families that underlie this whole approach.

This philosophy of community care underlies the recent changes proposed for nurse education by the United Kingdom Central Council. The *Report on Proposals for the Future of Community Education and Practice* (UKCC 1991), illustrates how health needs are closely related to social needs and shows how this should be reflected in the educational programmes provided for nurses working in the community. Health needs cannot be considered in isolation from social needs, or from the rôles of professionals who are themselves representatives of the communities they serve. The Report recommends that all nurses working in the community should undergo a shared core of preparation common to all practitioners, and that extra modules of learning be provided for specialist skills for the particular area of community practice. These developments are aimed at providing an integrated and more flexible approach to the health needs of the diverse and complex communities existing in British society today. Some of these complexities and the ways in which nurses are responding to them are illustrated below. For this discussion I have adopted the phrase 'community health care nurse', which is the Report's definition of:

' . . . nurses who have completed a specific post-registration preparation in order to provide a skilled nursing service to the community.'

(UKCC, 1991)

The concept of the sick rôle

In order to consider the kind of social world that is entered when professional help is sought, we need to give attention to the relationships between professionals and the public, and to examine the care they offer in the community. There are a number of possible models that could provide for such an examination. One example is the Health Belief Model developed by psychologists to predict and explain why individuals will or will not take advice or comply with medical regimens (Rosenstock, 1974). Although this model provides a useful guide to health behaviour in some circumstances, it becomes unnecessarily unwieldy when used across a diverse and complex range of behaviours (Wallston and Wallston, 1984), or as a framework in which to examine the rôles of patients and professionals. Social scientists have for many years gone beyond merely describing these relationships; by constructing models of the basic features, they have sought to provide a theoretical framework for deeper exploration and debate. Talcott Parsons was one of the first sociologists to address this issue, and as his work made a significant contribution to medical sociology; it is a useful starting point for the analysis of the relationships of concern to us.

Parson's model is not a description of how health professionals actually behave towards the sick, but a set of rules giving a structure for what he considered to be *ideal behaviour*. He stressed the importance of health for the smooth running of society, and the rules which he sees as governing the relationships, with their specification of rights and obligations on both sides, are to enable the sick person to be restored to normal function as soon as possible. The concept of the sick rôle which he developed (Parsons, 1951; p. 436–8), and in which the duties of the two parties are laid down, is seen as complementary to the rôle of the healer, and defines a rôle that may be played by anyone, regardless of status. It has four components. The first is that the sick person can claim exemption from normal work and family duties, the extent of the exemption being relative to the degree of illness. In the second place, the patient is not held responsible for his or her illness, and has a right to sympathy and support. Balancing these rights, however, are obligations and duties, and these constitute the remaining two components: the obligation to get well as quickly as possible, and the duty to co-operate with competent medical help in order to accomplish this end.

In Parsons' analysis the rôles of doctor and patient are seen as reciprocal, the former having rights and obligations as much as the latter. First, it is the duty of the doctor to act in the interest of the patient and not to be governed by self interest. Second, s/he must apply a high degree of skill and knowledge. Third s/he must be objective, emotionally detached and professional in his or her adoption of attitudes and modes of behaviour. So long as these requirements are fulfilled, doctors are entitled to a number of privileges. They enjoy considerable professional autonomy, and this places them in a powerful and influential position in society. They perform intimate examinations and have a right to personal information, all of which gives them a degree of authority *vis-à-vis* the patient.

Parsons' model refers then, not only to rights and obligations of the sick, but also to rights and obligations on the part of others involved with them. As such it provides a useful framework in which to consider the rôle of community health care nurses, who, whilst working closely with general practitioners, bear a distinct moral relation to their patients and families, as well as to the wider communities in which they practise.

Variations in the use of the sick rôle

In order to have illness legitimized and to be exempted from social obligations in our society it is necessary for patients to seek out medical help. Parsons attributes the causes of both physical and mental illness, in part at least, to the individual patient. He claims that in an attempt to avoid social pressures and responsibilities the individual seeks an escape through illness. However, because this is thought to take place largely at an unconscious level, it is not held by Parsons to entail any blame on the part of the sick person. Because of the high degree of 'motivatedness in illness' claimed by Parsons, he concludes that it may 'legitimately be regarded as a type of deviant behaviour' (Parsons, 1951; p. 285). This tendency to deviance is described as:

> 'A process of motivated action on the part of the actor . . . tending to deviate from the complementary expectations of conformity with common standards so far as these are relevant to the definition of his rôle.'
>
> (Parsons, 1951; p. 206)

Parsons goes on to suggest that because deviance tends to disrupt the social system, it presents problems of social control. It is therefore the function of medical practice not simply to bring patients back to health, but to act on individuals so as to restore them to their active place in society. In this way he viewed medical practice as a controller of social order, the patient being seen as a *passive* recipient of care, someone who is *acted on* by health professionals. The foundation upon which Parsons built his theory and model was thus paternalistic; the necessity of passivity and compliance on the part of the patient (the adoption of an almost child-like attitude) contrasting with the authority and control exerted by the doctor.

Research in the field of the relationships of the professionals with patients and clients has shown great differences between the very general rules attaching to the sick rôle and the way people in fact behave on particular occasions. There are infinitely many varieties and modifications of the rôle, and the differences in knowledge and experience amongst patients, carers and professionals can result in a clash of perspectives. These differences in perception, or systematic disagreements between doctors and patients, were studied by Cartwright (1967), who described a study in which as many as 26 per cent of general practitioners considered over half of all consultations to be concerned with matters of only minor importance. A later study by Bowling (1981) put the figure even higher, 54 per cent of doctors maintaining that triviality constituted a serious problem. On closer questioning it was found that emotional problems were the most frequent examples of trivia cited by doctors. Following this discovery, it was suggested that nurses might provide an answer to the problem, and that by being available in general practice settings, patients might choose to take their problems to them. On reporting this idea to the doctors involved, one general practitioner is quoted as saying:

'Nurses could do much more but we doctors tend to be very conservative. We complain of having too much work but we are very reluctant to delegate any of it.'

(Bowling, 1981)

It can be seen that community health care nurses can be an important additional resource. By offering patients a different, but complementary, type of consultation they can save doctors time; not by doing doctors' work, but by doing the work that many doctors do *not* do; namely, spending time on issues that are often perceived by doctors as only loosely related to health and illness. By giving explanations and by exploring different ways of achieving healthy life styles, nurses can *prevent* further complications arising and provide a positive contribution both to general practice and to the outcomes of consultations between doctors and their clients. This was shown to be the case in the Reading research project, where a very high rate of patient satisfaction with the nurse practitioner rôle was demonstrated: many patients found the nurse a good listener, easier than the doctor to talk to, and better at understanding and explaining (Salisbury and Tettersall, 1988). This work supports the observations made 3 years previously by Dr Halfden Mahler, director general of the World Health Organization, who said:

'Nurses will become resources to people rather than resources to physicians; they will become more active in educating people on health matters.'

(Mahler, 1985)

Mahler also gave several examples of very successful projects in which by far the greatest amount of advice and support was provided by nurses in their rôle as health educators. One such project was the Finnish Karelia project, which was highly successful in reducing the incidence of heart attacks in the population.

An important aspect of health and sickness behaviour, then, was omitted by Parsons in his analysis, and is often ignored by general practitioners. This is the fact that going to see health professionals is usually the *end process* of a complex system of health-seeking be-haviour (Mechanic, 1968; 268). Freidson (1961 and 1970) also directed attention to the process by which individuals seek medical help. The professional consultation takes place only *after* a series of 'consulta-tions' with significant lay groups. Freidson argues that it is this lay culture, not the doctor, that defines the meaning of illness in a social context:

'If a person perceives himself to be sick and in need of specialised help, he is likely to find support within his own cultural context only if he shows evidence of symptoms the others perceive to be illness, and if he interprets them the way others find plausible.'
(Freidson, 1970; p. 289)

There are clear implications here for health professionals, for if we are to influence patients and clients, we need to take account of their culture, social class, age and sex, as well as of their family members and the community in which we practise. The importance of accepting people as they are, and of taking account of the wider circumstances and constraints in which they live and work, is of major importance to the acceptability of, and compliance with, recommendations aimed at encouraging healthy living.

In his concept of the sick rôle Parsons also realised that the emo-tional connection between the doctor and the patient was an important aspect both of the diagnostic and of the therapeutic processes. He suggested that the doctor and the patient are committed to *severing* their relationships, rather than forming the more customary social connection in a stable style of interaction. The point of this reversal of the norm, Parsons argued, is that the sick rôle must be viewed as *temporary*, the whole aim of the exercise being to return the patient back into a social environment involving activism and obligation. Patients who constantly return to the doctor, and who are unable to withdraw from care, do not fit into Parsons' model, because it fails to take account of the fact that, for the chronically ill and disabled, the sick rôle becomes a more or less permanent state. Freidson (1970; p. 234) maintains that because chronically ill patients are unable to get well, the conditional legitimacy of Parsons' model is no longer valid. In other words, since the chronically sick patient is unable to get better, s/he is not able to enter the contract of striving to overcome the illness in return for certificates or prescriptions, but is expected to cope with long-term disability, and endure a sick rôle for life, often in social isolation.

Gallagher (1976; p. 209) also attacks Parsons' failure to account for chronic illness on the grounds of the inadequacy of the deviance model to account for the causes of illness. Since chronically ill patients have no prospect of returning to their former productivity and to normal social functioning, being given exemption from social obligations is an irrelevance. Gallagher also queries the obligation of the chronically long-term sick to co-operate with the doctor, since the doctor cannot deliver the patient from his or her dependency through the therapeutic use of social control mechanisms.

The community health care nurse's rôle with the chronically sick

It can be seen that for the case of chronically sick patients the relationship of the health professional and patient can be viewed differently from that suggested by Parsons' model. The importance of establishing mutual trust and of gaining the patient's confidence is obviously very desirable. Far from severing the relationship with the patient, it will be necessary to get to know the patient and his family well. The patient is no longer to be encouraged to be the passive beneficiary of medical care that Parsons' model suggests is necessary for reciprocity to take place. Instead, s/he will need to be encouraged to develop a high degree of autonomy and control over his or her condition, with many of the customary aspects of the doctor's rôle being delegated to the patient.

A satisfactory treatment of the chronically sick is not helped by a professional relationship that is asymmetrical, with the health professional being a rather dominant father or mother figure. Patients need to enter a contract of shared care, where it is accepted that information and knowledge about the illness is readily given, and where patients are encouraged to express their opinions about their progress and treatment. Studies such as that of Lewis and Resnick (1967) show how (in America) nurse practitioners hold successful sessions for the chronically sick. Patients claimed that they preferred these sessions to those held by doctors, the reasons given for their choice being generally concerned with the quality of the relationship; the nurses, they claimed, treated them as individuals, finding time to listen and to discuss their problems in full. In this way the nurses offered a different, and complementary, service to patients, enabling them to make use of services that they had felt diffident about calling upon in the past.

The community health care nurse's rôle in prevention

One of the basic tenets of Parsons' theory of the sick rôle is that the patient is blameless for his or her illness. Indeed, it is the very lack of responsibility for the illness that distinguishes the sick rôle from other forms of deviance, such as crime (Parsons, 1951; p. 440). Although it is still the case that patients are not held responsible for many illnesses, there are a growing number of conditions towards which the behaviour of the patient is considered to contribute. The effects on health of smoking, high-fat diet and lack of exercise have repeatedly been drawn to the attention of the public, with an accompanying readiness, particularly on the part of some politicians, to blame the sufferer for his or her complaint. In 1988 Edwina Curry, for instance, made it plain that she considered people in the North of England to be responsible for the higher incidence of heart disease through their refusal to accept the evidence of low-fat, high-fibre diets as being beneficial to health, and to change their eating habits accordingly. It has been argued, notably by Crawford (1977), that this kind of 'victim blaming' ignores the social and political influences of commercial and industrial origin that cause much of the unhealthy behaviour in society. A great deal of ill health is brought about by *collective* irresponsible behaviour result-ing in polluted air, water, and food supplies:

> 'Man is very rapidly becoming the cause of his own major reasons for death and disability through various errors of either omission or commission.'
>
> (James, 1968)

This is no doubt so. It would, for instance, be unwarranted to blame the individual consumer for illnesses consequent upon the improper preparation and handling of foodstuffs. However, as knowledge of the deleterious effects of certain forms of diet, and of ways of conducting one's life more generally, becomes more firmly established and more widely promulgated, it becomes increasingly more difficult to absolve the individual from all responsibility for the ill effects which an imprudent life style may bring in its wake.

The community health care nurse's rôle in health education

Nurse practitioners have a major responsibility in providing informa-tion to assist patients' understanding about issues affecting health, including the large number of present-day health problems which are behaviourally induced. Community health care nurses in particular are well placed to fulfil a valuable function in primary and secondary prevention. Parsons' model fails to account for this aspect of the health professional's work, although he does include aspects of health education which begin subsequent to hospital contact and which link to his conception of the sick rôle. His concern was with *tertiary* health education, with the management of illness and encouragement of compliance with medically approved regimes of treatment and advice. Parsons' focus once again takes for granted the authority of health professionals over patients and their relatives. His emphasis was on *resocialisation*, on trying to achieve a reversal in an established behaviour pattern which often results in the patients' being given a list of prohibitions by an authority figure. Such strategies have been seen to have only a very limited success rate, and the emphasis, particularly over the past decade, has changed. Whilst primary health education concentrates on creating and moulding value systems that invest in healthy life styles, and on leading individuals to behave in ways which avoid future ill-health, secondary health education focusses on halting or deferring health problems. This frequently involves motivating *well* individuals to use health-screening programmes and other prophylactic services, or to educate them in self-diagnosis techniques and to seek further help should this be necessary. Many of these services are not provided by general practitioners in person; instead they employ nurses to undertake such aspects of health work.

The research in 1987 of Greenfield, Stilwell and Drury showed how nurses working in general practice had attitudes and skills different from those of the doctors. Doctors are trained within an illness model where the emphasis is placed on diagnosing physical disease and giving treatment, often in the form of medication (Pitts and Vincent, 1989). Nurses, however, place more emphasis on practical care, advice, and health education; they can be seen to provide a *balance* between the rational scientific approach which seeks a remedy for an illness, and the approach which shows a greater involvement with the patient's personal needs, and more warmth, caring and sympathy (Gray, 1982). In providing an environment for health education these qualities are imperative, as patients will not attend sessions unless they feel welcome, and will not learn or be motivated to try new approaches or forms of behaviour unless they are given support and encouragement.

In a study by Cartwright and Anderson (1981) less than a third of all patients said that they would feel able to ask their general practitioner for help with a personal problem, and various studies show that patients perceive nurses as more approachable than doctors and will more readily seek their help with intimate matters. In particular, in a study by Hull and Hull (1984), 47 per cent of the women interviewed found it difficult to tell the doctor why they had attended the surgery. The same study showed that a large proportion of patients were dissatisfied with the period of time that their general practitioners were prepared to spend with them. Another study by Lazare and colleagues found that 30 per cent of the patients whom they questioned had a 'hidden agenda' for the visit that was not elicited, whilst many other patients were left feeling dissatisfied with the interview. The researchers concluded that:

'Conflict is inevitable in the vast majority of encounters.'
(Lazare *et. al.*, 1979; p. 162)

Most of this conflict is due, at least in part, to the brevity of consultations, which is seen as a major constraint in general practice. Whilst one answer might be to reduce the numbers on a doctor's list, another is to develop and extend the rôles of community health care nurses. A research study carried out in Reading (Salisbury and Tettersell, 1988) showed that patients found very high levels of satisfaction with the care provided by a nurse practising an extended rôle. Patients reported that they felt that the nurse had encouraged them to participate, that she appeared unhurried, and had been prepared to listen to them and treat them as individuals. Undoubtedly the amount of time the nurse gave to each consultation influenced the patients' perceptions of the quality of the service, as it allowed for a relationship to develop between nurse and patient. Adopting this style of consultation facilitates the 'shared care' ethic and encourages patients to take responsibility for reviewing their lifestyles and adapting them where necessary.

Mental illness and the sick rôle

In the sociology of mental health, the dominant paradigm for the explanation of mental illness has been labelling theory. Medical sociology adopted a range of models which had been designed initially for the explanation of deviance, because it followed the Parsonian model which approached sickness as a form of social deviance. Diverse forms of behaviour are labelled deviant, not because they share any uniform themes or experiences, but because they are defined as such by powerful, influential or significant social groups which are important in shaping public opinion. People who are labelled as deviant suffer stigmatization which excludes them from normal social interactions; this in turn reinforces their original behaviour because alternative lifestyles and careers are no longer available to them. This approach is aptly summarized by Cooley (1902) who developed the theory of the 'looking-glass self'. He suggested that people become deviant or mentally ill when they cease to receive positive definitions of themselves from their primary social groups.

A piece of research that helps to illustrate these effects was undertaken in 1973 by Rosenhan. In this study nine subjects agreed to present themselves at a psychiatric hospital complaining of hearing voices. Once they had been admitted they behaved normally, experiencing no further problems and telling staff that they felt well. Although the periods over which they were held differed, the average stay was 19 days. During this time they reported disturbing interactions with members of staff. They gave examples of staff ignoring their requests, talking over them and treating them as incompetent and insane. Labelling can thus be seen as a powerful force in social relations and may be a reason why many mentally ill patients refuse to adopt a sick rôle lifestyle.

The permanent sick rôle lifestyle

Replying to Parsons' sick rôle model, Merton (1957; pp. 112–26) suggested that in some instances sickness could become a permanent solution to the structural contradictions of contemporary society. An individual might gain important secondary benefits from being sick, avoiding responsibilities and retreating from the demands of social pressures. A minority of individuals, he argued, feel excluded from our Western industrialist society, based as it is on an activist culture and a norm of achievement, and may wish to manipulate the means or ends of that culture for illegitimate purposes. Merton suggests that drug addiction would be one such example of this kind of retreatism, representing a deviant but permanent adaptation to the social structure. Clearly this situation could be seen to lead to conflicts in the health professional/patient relationship, between the health worker's commitment to helping the patient to get well, and the patient's commitment to a sick rôle lifestyle.

In circumstances like these, where the conventional sick rôle model has been abolished, patients may not receive any treatment at all. Barbara Burke-Masters (1983) has described how homeless and destitute people were denied primary health care and therefore other health services which normally follow via the referral system. Griffiths (1981) had previously claimed that thousands of people, living rough or in hotels, have, in effect, no access to a local doctor. The reason for this is that general practitioners do not receive payment for registering as a permanent patient anyone of no fixed abode, and, although they can claim payment if they register patients as temporary residents, they are in practice very reluctant to do so.

Jeffery (1984) showed how such patients, who did not conform to the sick rôle, were labelled as 'bad' and treated with animosity by many doctors. These patients broke the rules of the doctor/patient relationship and the expectations of reciprocity in giving and receiving treatment. In the first place they were regarded as being responsible for their own illnesses and conditions. Secondly, they refused to be restricted in their daily activities or to cooperate with doctors in their treatment. Thirdly, the patients failed to see their conditions as undesirable. Many preferred this nomadic kind of lifestyle and were not motivated to make the changes advocated by medical practitioners. In all these aspects these patients failed to fit into Parsons' model by refusing to adopt the customary rights and obligations allotted to the sick rôle. In 1980 Burke–Masters began working on a project to provide medical/nursing care to vagrant alcoholics. She found that her patients had multiple problems and that in order to respond to their needs she needed to extend her rôle and become an autonomous practitioner with greater powers of diagnosis, treatment and referral. After a number of setbacks she was able to act as a link worker and put patients into direct contact with the treatment and specialist help that they so desperately needed.

The sick rôle and stigmatization

One reason why these patients may refuse to adopt a sick rôle lifestyle is because, as we have remarked, all sickness carries a certain stigma, and so rather than being made better by adopting a sick rôle, matters can actually be made worse. Erikson (1957) saw this contradiction when Parsons' model was applied to psychiatric illness. If a mentally ill person seeks professional help, it may also result in stigmatization, so that social withdrawal is legitimized by the doctor during an acute phase of illness, but the normal medical and social obligation to get well and return to usual duties is replaced by an obligation to remain sick which is established for the patient, often as a result of what is viewed as his or her anti-social behaviour. Paradoxically, however, there is often an element of personal responsibility assumed, particularly by the public, with the expectation that the patient should work hard to get better and fit back into the conventional mould. The patient may be seen as 'opting out' by assuming the sick rôle, and withdrawal from work and social duties may be refused.

Medical practice is seen as being both important and influential in shaping public opinion. The ways in which health professionals define, explain, and develop systems of treatment for the mentally sick contribute towards the common public consciousness of mental illness. Differences in the rates of such illness experienced by different social groups and classes are directly associated with the prevalence of stressful events such as loss and bereavement, unemployment and poverty, and the vulnerability factors of a particular individual such as age, social class, ethnic minority and sex. It has been shown that if an individual is experiencing a high level of stress and has a high personal vulnerability score s/he is likely to need additional support from his or her friends and community:

'The greater the social support that an individual receives, in the form of closer relations with family members, kin, friends, acquaintances, co-workers, and the larger community, the less likely it is that the individual will experience illness.'

(Lin *et. al.*, 1979; p. 109)

It has been shown (Levine *et. al.*, 1978) that nurses are found to be very approachable by patients with a wide variety of problems. By showing acceptance of patients experiencing stress or psychiatric difficulties, and by giving information to relatives in order to equip them to care for patients, community health care nurses can again provide a valuable link between patients and their carers as well as helping to dispel some of the negative attitudes that exist in society today.

The sick rôle and the elderly

Another weakness in Parsons' model is that illness is not the only legitimate cause of withdrawal from work and social responsibilities. Ageing, with the slow onset of disability and withdrawal from social rôles, could not be regarded as a genuine sick rôle. If it was to be viewed in this light, then retirement could be seen as a form of transference of an individual to a permanent sick rôle. This is an important conception, as the psychological impact of retirement, loss of status, bereavement and the imagined stigma of being dependent upon society, pose a threat to the physical and mental health of the elderly. Many elderly patients are often willing to enter the sick rôle and to accept disease and disability as being an integral part of ageing. This was confirmed by the work of Brocklehurst (1975) who showed that many elderly people ignore the signs and symptoms of disease because they believe that there is no treatment or cure, and that sickness and disability in old age are inevitable.

With the proportion of elderly people increasing in the population, the rôle of community health care nurses needs to expand. Opportunities exist in preventive work to minimize the effects of degenerative diseases and to prevent complications arising from ignorance or increased isolation.

In her work in rural Scotland, for example, Doreen Restall (Stilwell *et. al.*, 1988) felt that many of the problems expressed by elderly patients could have been dealt with by the nurses 'giving simple advice education and treatment'. The research study, which was designed to screen for and to identify depression in the elderly, covered physical, social, and environmental aspects of health. Although 17 per cent of the sample were reported as having unmet health needs, many attributed their health problems to their age, and others considered that the nature of their problems was too trivial to take to their general practitioner. Following this experience Restall decided to review and extend her rôle, as she felt that in order to prevent further deterioration in her patients' conditions she needed to be more available for both patients and their relatives:

> 'To provide an alternative consultative pattern (for) the public, particularly to meet the needs of those who would not normally attend the general practitioner with so called "trivial" or minor illnesses. The nurse practitioner's rôle includes assessment, problem-solving, teaching, counselling and health education. The nurse practitioner can evaluate, screen, identify and assist to identify illness and render appropriate treatment where necessary, or refer to the general practitioner.'
>
> (Stilwell, *et. al.*, 1988)

The importance of the nurse's rôle in prevention and in caring for the elderly was acknowledged in the recent Government White Paper, *Working for Patients* (DHSS, 1989). For nurses to provide the kind of service that is now needed in the community, it will be necessary to grant them greater autonomy. Littlewood (1989) has suggested that nurses are much better placed than doctors to understand and deal with the problems of the elderly. She describes the crucial rôle of nursing in assessing and managing the health problems encountered in old age. In particular, the 'quick fix' approach of doctors during their consultations is either inappropriate or of little benefit. The elderly need to be given time to express themselves and nurses are often seen as more approachable and more prepared to listen to the accounts which old people give of what it is that gives meaning to their lives. Littlewood therefore sees the nurse as the health professional best placed to 'negotiate between the goals of the doctor . . . and the goals of the patient' (Littlewood, 1989; pp. 221–9).

This nursing practice is taken for granted in the hospital setting where nurses spend time with patients discussing interventions and treatments recommended by the doctors. Among the elderly this is particularly the case, with the patients needing to go over possible diagnostic and therapeutic procedures several times, reflecting on what has been said, and then asking for further explanation and information. Where precise compliance is an important issue, as in the case of prescribed drugs, patient understanding and cooperation is essential for the treatment to be effective. The utility of counselling in guarding against medication errors by elderly patients was recorded by MacDonald *et. al.* (1977). The researchers found that counselled patients made under one third of the errors committed by uncounselled patients, and that counselling was almost as effective in improving compliance even when the patient was poorly orientated. It can be seen that spending time with patients is not simply a luxury service, but that it can have a major impact on the understanding of patients and on their ability to comply, and therefore on the quality of their life in old age.

Rôle negotiation: the challenge to change

As we have seen, Parsons' model draws attention to the contract entered into by patients and their doctors. In the *ideal relationship* described by Parsons the patient is seen as a submissive agent accepting and acting upon the doctor's prescriptive counsel. Indeed, the definition of a good professional relationship used to be one in which health professionals were able to distance themselves from their patients and not become personally involved with the problems experienced by the client. The emphasis was on seeking a physical cause to a problem and finding a cure, thus enabling the patient to return to normal social functioning. Criticising Parson's idealized view of the doctor/patient relationship, Freidson (1961) suggests that nurses are often required to interpret comments and instructions to patients following consultations with doctors. Porter (1988) and Brearley (1990), taking the argument further, discuss the rôle of the nurse as patient advocate. Salvage (1987) suggests that, since nurses are the main providers of care, support, and information, they are in the best position to fulfil the rôle of advocate and help the powerless in their struggle against the powerful. As we have seen in this chapter, nurses working among the homeless, the elderly, and other disadvantaged groups have many opportunities to act as advocates for their patients.

One of the most important findings to emerge from this exploration of the relationships between the public and health professionals is that the *nature* and *quality* of these interactions has considerable influence on patient satisfaction. Since Parsons first introduced his model in the 1950s, and particularly over the last decade, the levels of satisfaction experienced by patients following medical consultations have declined. One major reason for this decline is that patients have become more knowledgeable about health matters (Cartwright and Anderson, 1981), and are therefore more able to criticise the advice they are given. Perhaps more important for our discussion of the changing rôle of nurses in the community is the research that highlights the extent to which patients have become critical of the *style* of these communications (Sachs, 1983). This perhaps reflects a more critical approach to human relationships to be found more generally in present-day society. Whereas in the past people would not feel that it was their place to be critical of such authoritative figures as doctors or nursing sisters, they nowadays evince a greater readiness to express dissatisfaction.

It is in this area of patient dissatisfaction that the challenge to overhaul our practice lies, and in so far as this dissatisfaction is justified, it is our responsibility to seek ways to make good the deficiencies in the present system. As we have noted, not all patients who attend the surgery are sick; they attend with a variety of complaints that often mask underlying problems. Patients are therefore motivated to label themselves as sick and to enter the sick rôle in order to get help, there being nowhere else for them to turn. Many of these patients present to the doctor with vague symptoms, or will return to the surgery again and again, because treatment is not giving them the help they need. Such consultations are, as we have seen, highly frustrating for the doctor, and undesirable in economic terms, as expensive drugs may be tried, followed by referrals to hospitals for costly diagnostic procedures.

Community health care nurses can offer an alternative consultative service to patients by encouraging them to attend with a view to talking over their lifestyles as well as their symptoms. In consequence, patients may choose not to enter the sick rôle but to continue with their normal social functions with professional support. This shift of emphasis towards prevention effects a radical reversal of the usual conception of the nurse's rôle. Not only should the approach proposed contribute to a broadening of choice and a lessening of dissatisfaction, but it should also lead to significant financial savings.

The requirement to be able to understand and to meet the needs of patients draws on the traditional qualities of the nursing profession. The ability of nurses to *care* and to offer open access for consultations on non-medical as well as on medical matters is becoming increasingly important. As we saw in the research undertaken in the Birmingham study (Drury, Greenfield, Stilwell and Hull, 1988), patients *chose* to see the nurse for counselling, and social and emotional problems as well as for health information. Support in times of emotional upheaval is more readily sought from nurses, whereas doctors are seen as 'rational, scientific, unemotional and uninvolved'. Patients also were keen to see the nurse over health education and screening procedures.

Today's image of community nurses and their rôle in health education is portrayed in policy proposals as one in which they help patients to help themselves. The form of relationship which would be most conducive to this end would be one similar to that described by Szasz and Hollender (1956) as the 'mutual participation' type. This concept has gone hand in hand with the use of an active negotiation process which increases client and family participation, and enhances personal decision-making and responsibility. Operating this model within traditional structures involves a shifting of power alignments away from professional domination towards an interdependence of shared power and of the pursuit of common goals.

In this respect Parsons' theory does not allow for the vision needed in health care in the 1990s. It sees health in terms of getting people back to a stage where they can continue to fulfil social obligations and rôles – in other words to carry on *as they did before*. For many this rôle may be precisely the cause of their distress, whether it involves difficulties at home or in the workplace, or simply an unfulfilling and monotonous lifestyle. For such people there is an urgent need to explore patterns of behaviour or lifestyles with a view to bringing about positive change and improvement, and to giving them a sense of wholeness and well-being.

As individuals assume greater responsibility for their own lives, so too must community health care nurses become increasingly accountable for providing services designed to meet the needs of the population they serve. Historically, health professionals have decided what services they wish to provide, with minimal attention to what the public wants or feels it needs. With the help of Government legislation, this trend is changing. The increased levels of knowledge and self-responsibility among clients necessitates a receptiveness among health professionals to deliver care that effectively and efficiently meets the needs of consumers. Health care should be offered to patients on equal terms; the hierarchical structure is now outmoded and unacceptable, both towards patients and within the primary health care team. It is also the case that our economy can no longer support a 'fix-it' orientation to health, whereby people live as they choose and seek health care to repair the ravages to their bodies consequent upon unhealthy lifestyles.

In order to be effective, community health care nurses adopt a problem-solving approach to meet client needs. This means that assessment, planning, implementation and evaluation comprise a viable way to examine, critique, and where necessary modify the health care system which they provide. To date the nursing process has been utilized effectively with individuals and families; now it needs to be extended for use in the entire community. This framework will provide a structure in which nurses can act as agents for change in the system in which nursing care is offered.

References

Bowling, A. (1981). *Delegation in General Practice. A study of Doctors and Nurses*. Tavistock, London.

Brearley, S. (1990). *Patient Participation: The Literature*. Royal College of Nursing, London.

Brocklehurst, J. C. (1975). *Geriatric Care in Advanced Societies*. Blackburn Times Press, Blackburn.

Burke-Masters, B. (1983). Pseudo tags won't stick. *Doctor*, October 13, 1953.

Cartwright, A. (1976). *Patients and Their Doctors*. Routledge and Kegan Paul, London.

Cartwright, A. and Anderson R. (1981). *General Practice Revisited*. Tavistock, London.

Cooley, C. H. (1902). *Human Nature and the Social Order*. Scribners, New York.

Crawford, R. (1977). Ideology and politics of victim blaming. *International Journal of Health Services*, **7(4)**, 663–80.

Drury, M., Greenfield, S., Stilwell, B. and Hull, F. (1988). A nurse practitioner in general practice: patient perceptions and expectations. *Journal of the Royal College of General Practitioners*, **38**, 503–5.

Erikson, K. (1957). Patient rôle and uncertainty: A dilemma of the mentally ill. *Psychiatry*, **20**, 263–74.

Freidson, E. (1961). *Patients' Views of Medical Practice*. Russell Sage Foundation, New York.

Freidson, E. (1970). *Profession of Medicine*. Dodd Mead, New York.

Gallagher, E. B. (1976). Lines of reconstruction and extension in the Parsonian sociology of illness. *Social Science and Medicine*, **10**, 207–18.

Gray, J. (1982). The effect of the doctor's sex on the doctor–patient relationship. *Journal of the Royal College of General Practitioners*, **38**, 503–5.

Greenfield, S., Stilwell, B. and Drury M. (1987) Practice nurses: social and occupational characteristics. *Journal of the Royal College of General Practitioners*, **37**, 341–5.

Griffiths, R. (1981). *Introduction to the Report of the Conference Arranged by the Association of Community Health Councils for England and Wales: The Campaign for the Homeless and Rootless*. ACHEW, London.

Hull, F. M. and Hull, F. S. (1984). Time and the general practitioner: the patient's view. *Journal of the Royal College of General Practitioners*, **34**, 71–5.

James, G. (1968). Human Potential in a Dynamic Environment. *School Health Education Study*, Washington DC.

Jeffrey, R. (1984). Normal rubbish: deviant patients in casualty departments, *Health and Disease: A Reader*. Open University Press, Milton Keynes.

Lazare, A. *et. al.* (1979). A negotiated approach to the clinical encounter, *Outpatient Psychiatry*. Williams and Williams, Baltimore.

Lewis, C. and Resnick, B. (1967). Nurse clinics and progressive ambulatory care. *New England Journal of Medicine*, **277**, 1236–41.

Levine, S. *et. al.* (1978). The sick rôle: assessment and overview. *The Annual Review of Sociology*, **4**, 317–43.

Littlewood, J. (1989). A model for nursing using anthropological literature. *International Journal of Nursing Studies*, **26**, 221–9.

Macdonald, E., Macdonald, J. and Phoenix, M. (1977). Improving drug compliance after hospital discharge. *British Medical Journal*, **2**, 618–21.

Mahler, H. (1985). Nurses Lead the Way. *WHO Features* No. 97.

Mechanic, D. (1968). *Medical Sociology*. The Free Press, New York.

Merton, R. K. (1957). *Social Theory and Social Structure*. The Free Press, Glencoe, Illinois.

Parsons, T. (1951). *The Social System*. Routledge & Kegan Paul, London.

Pitts, J. (1989). What influences doctors' prescribing? *Journal of the Royal College of General Practitioners*, **39**, 319.

Porter, S. (1988). Siding with the system. *Nursing Times*, **84(41)**, 30–1.

Restall, D. (1988). Nurse practitioners in British general practice, In *The Nurse in Family Practice*, pp. 75–76. A. Bowling and B. Stilwell (Eds). Scutari, London.

Rosenhall, D. (1973). On being sane in insane places. *Science*, **179**, 250–8.

Rosenstock, I. M. (1974). The health belief model and preventive health behaviour. *Health Education Monographs*, **2**, 354–86.

Sachs, H. (1983). Rethinking general practice. *Dilemmas in Primary Care*. Tavistock, London.

Salisbury, C. and Tettersall, M. (1988). Comparison of the work of a nurse practitioner with that of a general practitioner. *Journal of the Royal College of General Practitioners*, **38**, 314–16.

Salvage, J. (1987). Whose side are you on? *Senior Nurse* **6(2)**, 20–1.

Stilwell, B., Restall, D. and Burke-Masters, B. (1988). Nurse practitioners in British general practice. In *The Nurse in Family Practice*. A. Bowling and B. Stilwell (Eds), pp. 69–82. Scutari, London.

Szasz, T. S. and Hollender, M. H. (1956). A contribution to the philosophy of medicine: the basic models of the doctor-patient relationship. *Archives of Internal Medicine*, **97**, 585–92.

United Kingdom Central Council for Nursing, Midwifery and Health Visiting (1991). Report on Proposals for the Future of Community Education and Practice.

Wallston, B. S. and Wallston, K. A. (1984) Social psychological models of health and behaviour: an examination and integration. In *Handbook of Psychology and Health*, Vol 4, pp. 23–53. A. Baum, S. E. Singer and J. Singer (Eds), Erlbaum, Hillsdale, N.J.

Suggested further reading

Brown, P. (1989). *Perspectives in Medical Sociology*. Wadsworth, California.

George, J. B. (Ed), (1985). *Nursing Series: The Base for Professional Nursing Practice*. Prentice Hall, London.

Niven, N. (1989). *Health Psychology: An Introduction for Nurses and other Health Care Professionals*. Churchill Livingstone, London.

Redman, B. K. (1988). *The Process of Patient Education*. Mosby Press, Washington.

Turner, B. S. (1987). *Medical Power and Social Knowledge*. Sage Publications, London.

4 Rethinking the nursing process

The notion of planned individualised patient care as a systematic process has been a part of British nursing since the mid-1970s. However, much of the empirical evidence to date demonstrates that more than a decade since its introduction, the nursing process is misunderstood and largely rejected by nurses as a meaningful, practical tool for organising patient care. Many of the arguments against the nursing process, however, are aimed at the documentation of patient care and little distinction has been made between the process and its documentation.

This chapter will focus on rethinking what the nursing process is and what it is not. In many senses, the ideas and concepts put forward in many of the other chapters in this book are ideas and concepts which influence our understanding of the nursing process. In a sense, then, attempts will be made to incorporate such notions as values, philosophies of care, models of nursing, quality assurance and the concept of caring into new understandings of the nursing process.

Values and philosophies of care

In any discussion about values and philosophies of care, certain assumptions need to be made. In the case of the nursing process, the assumption is made that nursing process – the systematic approach to planning and giving care – is a good thing and that planning care through this systematic approach is potentially an effective way of being very clear about what care we wish to give and why.

The basis for this assumption is another assumption: that quality patient care is given through well thought-out, justified decisions, the effects of which can be measured against agreed goals or aims of care.

The nursing process then is about forming appropriate relationships with patients, collecting information as the basis for decision-making, using the information to clarify needs for care and priorities, exploring the range of care options available to meet care needs, making professional judgements about which options to choose, taking action and evaluating the effectiveness of the choice of action.

What has just been described is a decision-making process for nursing, and this is what the nursing process is – congruent with the notion of the nurse as a 'knowledgeable doer' as described by the United Kingdom Central Council for Nursing, Midwifery and Health Visiting (1986) and as a decision-making process, the nursing process is a way of being very clear about what nurses are doing as they prescribe and give care and why. It enables nurses to justify or account for any of their nursing actions and more importantly, enables nurses to re-think their choice of action as they measure the effectiveness of the care they give.

There is a close relationship between this decision-making process and the whole area of standard setting and monitoring the quality of the care we give. Donabedian (1969) described a structure-process-outcome approach to standards of care (*see* Chapter 7) and certain parallels between the Donabedian model and the nursing process can be drawn. Process standards describe the process of nursing which is to count as acceptable practice. Using the nursing process to achieve desired outcomes enables nurses to make predictive statements about what they expect their care to achieve. In accounting for their nursing actions nurses measure the extent to which the process of their nursing has achieved the desired outcomes. In other words, nurses need to get the process right to have any chance of getting the desired outcome.

However, much of the evidence shows that nursing has not got the process of nursing right. If this is so, then an examination of what has gone wrong in the use of the nursing process may be necessary. Possible explanations for the failure of this process are offered here.

Firstly, one explanation might be that the nursing process is, in itself, wrong/inappropriate/ineffective. It is hard to conceive that such a rational decision-making system could be inherently wrong. Nurses need to have systems by which decisions are made. Historical rationale for nursing actions like 'we've always done it this way' or 'Sister (or Doctor) told me to do this', have little place in the professional world of the 'knowledgeable doer' or the accountable practitioner (United Kingdom Central Council for Nursing, Midwifery and Health Visiting, 1984). Therefore, other explanations as to why the nursing process has failed must be sought.

A new way of thinking imposed on an old way of acting

An eminent nurse once stood up at a conference on the nursing process and made a statement that the nursing process was the most sophistic-ated form of task allocation. This could easily be so. One of the fundamental reasons for the apparent lack of success in implementing the nursing process is that historically, nursing has been perceived and carried out as a series of tasks. Whether nurses were given lists of tasks to carry out (the dressings, the blanket baths, the bed-pan rounds and so forth) or whether nurses are allocated patients, nursing care is still commonly practised as tasks. The nurse who is allocated Mrs Smith in bed three tends largely to identify tasks to be carried out on or for or with Mrs Smith. If the nursing process is superimposed onto this historical way of practising nursing, the stages in the nursing process also become tasks to do; e.g., the task of taking a case history, of writing a care plan, of updating the care plan, and so forth. Whereas the tasks of giving direct patient care are seen as legitimate in the eyes of most nurses, the tasks of writing documents are seen to have little value – they are extra tasks to do which keep nurses away from giving direct patient care. So long as the nursing process is seen as a system superimposed onto old ways of viewing nursing, then nursing process will continue to be additional tasks which are given less value than direct care giving tasks.

Before the nursing process can assume a different meaning to nurses, what is needed is a fundamental shift in the way nurses view nursing and nursing care. So long as nurses continue to perceive their work as tasks/procedures to carry out, then so too will nursing process join that long list of nursing tasks.

If, however, a shift took place in how nurses defined nursing, then nursing process, too, would assume a different place in the way we view our nursing work. If, for example, nursing were to be viewed by nurses as a dynamic process of thinking, doing and being, then the nursing process would also be seen as a dynamic process of thinking, doing and being. The *thinking* part of nursing process is the part of nursing which collects information, explores relationships between information, examines options and makes professional decisions about care. The *doing* part of the nursing process is the giving of care, putting into action the thinking and decisions. The *being* part of the nursing process is the forming of interpersonal relationships between nurse and patient, without which, the *thinking* and *doing* parts become tasks.

Unless nurses re-think their perceptions and definitions of what nursing is, then the nursing process will remain as tasks to be carried out. Tasks are about products. Process is about how nurses make decisions, plan, think, feel, and are, as they aim to reach an outcome.

In most nursing settings if one is asked, 'Are you using the nursing process?' the response tends to be to show the care plan (product). Judgement about whether or not a ward/unit is 'using the nursing process' is made on production of the product (the care plan). However, many clinical areas have beautiful products (care plans) but the ethos of nursing process as a dynamic decision-making process of thinking, doing and being is absent. Conversely, there are clinical areas which have no sign of the product (the care plans) but where the ethos of nursing is a dynamic decision-making process of thinking, doing and being, where nurses know why they've made the care decisions they have made and can account for their actions through evaluation of patient outcomes.

So what is the difference between the ethos and practice of the nursing process and the production of a written care plan? The answer to this, if such an answer is possible, requires further examination of the definition of nursing process itself. The traditional definition of the nursing process is that it is a systematic approach to nursing care which has four (or sometimes more) stages: assessing, planning, implementing, and evaluating (Yura and Walsh: 1983).

However, in terms of examining the nursing process as a dynamic decision-making process of thinking, doing and being, another definition might be offered; that the nursing process is a particular set of values and beliefs which is put into practice through nursing.

The words which have been used to describe the value system behind nursing process are important. The literature on nursing process abounds with phrases like, 'the rights of patients to be treated as unique and autonomous individuals,' 'holistic care,' 'individualised care,' and so forth. If this is the value system underpinning nursing process then nurses need to ask themselves some very serious questions about what needs to be a primary feature of their nursing in order to put this value system into practice. If the real goal of nursing is to put into practice this humanistic value system then assessment of patients becomes more than gathering information and recording it on a nursing history sheet. Instead, assessment is about forming a relationship with a person, getting to know him as a person and allowing him to get to know the nurse. Through this relationship, information will come but the focus of assessment in the new definition of nursing process is the building of the relationship. Therefore, the assessment skills required to be used by nurses include the skills of initiating and building relationships, trust-building, self-disclosure and so forth (Marks-Maran, 1988). Through the relationship, meaningful information is then obtained.

As nurses move away from the old tasks of the nursing process like the task of taking a history, and move towards person-to-person relationship-building as the basis for assessment, a number of things happen. Firstly, the shift in emphasis is away from filling in a form and moves instead to an emphasis on getting to know someone as a person. Secondly, the approach moves from, 'Good morning, Mrs Smith. I'd like to get some information from you in order to best plan your care,' and moves to, 'Good morning, Mrs Smith, I'm going to be looking after you today. Let's get to know each other a little better.'

Process is a two way dynamic with information being shared between both parties rather than one person getting information from another. The logical follow-on from this is the notion that part of the underlying ethos of nursing process is that of partnership. Assessment of patients should reflect this ethos of partnership. From a teaching point of view, teaching nursing process is firstly about helping students clarify their values and beliefs about nursing and about people, and secondly, about helping the students explore the concepts associated with nursing process which are partnership, people-centredness, respect for individuality, autonomy, dignity and so forth. The kind of skills our nursing programmes must provide to help nurses to practise within the new definition of nursing process are skills of listening, sharing, caring for self, talking with patients, using our intuition and putting partnership into practice. In other words, assessment skills are the same as the skills of building relationships and personal growth and development. So long as nursing stays locked into a definition of assessment which is about the task of filling in a nursing history, so too will nursing be locked into the product and not the process.

So far, the discussion has focussed on initial assessment of patients. Since assessment is an ongoing and recurring process, re-assessment is also about a one-to-one relationship between nurse and patient. The skills nurses need to use are those involved in discussing with patients how they (the patients) feel their care is progressing, what their perception of their progress is, and whether they believe that their own personal goals are being achieved. It is a time of sharing the nurse's perception of patient progress with the patient's own perception of his progress.

Using assessment information

The purpose of building a caring relationship with a patient ultimately is to get to know each other better and through this, to allow information to be shared and clarified in order to plan future nursing care. Information which the nurse receives from the patient might be:

- facts
- thoughts
- feelings expressed by patients
- feeling not explicitly expressed but demonstrated non-verbally

Following every assessment interview in our re-defined nursing process, the nurse should take time to reflect on the interview. Perhaps the following questions might assist in this:

1. What facts have been gained which I need to act on?
2. What are the patient's thoughts on his illness/admission/treatment/ progress?
3. What feelings has he shared with me and how can I act on this information?
4. What non-verbal cues did I notice? Have I checked out with the patient that I am interpreting his non-verbal messages accurately? How am I going to act on this information?
5. What facts do I know about his illness/operation/treatment which will influence the care that I decide to give? What information do I

need to share with him to enable him to be making informed decisions?

6. What is my intuition telling me about this person?

From this, the nurse makes certain decisions, albeit tentative, about the patient's need for care and what the priorities of care might be. As we re-think nursing process, there is also an important step between the nurse deciding the care that is needed and the nurse actually beginning to give that care. The step is this; in a two-way partnership relationship which is what the nursing process is, the nurse needs to check out with the patient that her (the nurse's) perception of needs and priorities is the same as the patient's perception. This is done through an interaction which may begin like this:

> 'Well, Mrs Smith, looking at the things we've been talking about, I've got the feeling that x, y and z are the most important things that I should be helping you sort out. How does this sound to you?'

It may also be appropriate for the nurse to give the patient any factual information about their illness, operation and treatment to enable the patient to understand how the nurse came to that decision about priorities.

There is a two-fold process going on at this point; the first is that the nurse is making connections between various pieces of information. This process of connecting pieces of assessment information to draw conclusions is referred to as a *nursing diagnosis* in the American nursing literature. Secondly, as an integral part of the relationship between nurse and patient, the nurse is checking out her perceptions and conclusions with the patient in order to agree common goals and share their understanding of care needs. This is an important part of the new understanding of the nursing process if we are to act on the values we hold about partnership in decision-making.

In summary then, using assessment information helps the nurse to clarify with the patient mutually agreed issues of importance so that both parties are working to the same set of priorities, perceptions and expectations. Historically, nurses have had more knowledge of the physiological priorities, potential problems arising from illness or treatment, and placed high priority on these. As we move to partnerships with patients, however, it is they who are more knowledgeable of the effects which their illness/treatment/operation is having on their self-concept, their role, and on their relationships with their loved ones. To place greater importance on the nurse's agenda of priorities negates the notion that it is only the patient who is in a position to determine what is of importance to him. The function of partnership nursing is to enable patients to have the right information so that they can determine what is to count as being of importance to them.

Planning and giving care

Following the establishment of a person-to-person relationship between nurse and patient, sharing of assessment information gained through that relationship, making relationships between the various pieces of assessment information, and then agreeing perceptions and priorities for care, the nurse is then in a knowledgeable position to make decisions about the nature of the nursing care she intends to prescribe. Wherever possible the nurse will look to available research findings to identify a course of nursing action most appropriate to a particular patient problem or need. In the absence of available research, empirical knowledge or theory will influence nursing care decisions. In any event, there may be a number of nursing options available to a nurse in any given situation. The nurse will choose from the available options, always mindful that in exercising professional judgement and in making nursing decisions, she is able to justify her choice of action at the time the decision is made. Part of the decision will involve identifying what effect she expects her nursing action to have on the patient and when and how she, and the patient, should be able to determine whether the decision taken is having its positive effect on patient progress. Some sort of measurable statement should be identified in order that some form of evaluation of care can take place against this measurable statement. Whatever nursing care is prescribed the nurse should be able to justify that decision with reference to theory, research, or in the absence of these, reasoned empirical evidence.

Evaluation

Evaluation of care and the documentation of that evaluation are two areas within the nursing process which have caused major problems for nurses. Although it is tempting to offer reasons why this difficulty has been encountered, it might be more appropriate to examine how evaluation of care might be made more meaningful for nurses and at the same time, be less daunting.

Evaluation of care is part of quality assurance. It is a way of demonstrating that our care decisions were appropriate and serves as a means by which we, and our patients, can judge the effectiveness of the care we offer. However, meaningful objective evaluation is only possible when there is a shared understanding of what the care was attempting to achieve in the first place. It comes as no surprise that, along with evaluation of care, nurses have also found it difficult to set goals in measurable terms. Yet without clearly identified, measureable goals shared with our patients, it becomes virtually impossible to make a meaningful professional judgement as to the success of nursing care interventions.

It is clear that evaluation of nursing is directly linked to goal setting. Setting goals with patients provide statements, in measurable terms, of what we expect the outcomes of our care to be. Unless nurses make these explicit statements of what they expect their care to specifically achieve, and by when, there are no yardsticks against which to measure the success of our nursing decisions.

Models of nursing and the nursing process

The nursing literature has much to offer about the relationship between models of nursing and the nursing process (George, 1985; Aggleton and Chalmers, 1986; Hunt and Marks-Maran, 1986). Despite the absence of research into the effectiveness of nursing models, one thing has become clear to many practitioners; nursing process on its own merely implies that it is a good thing to assess, plan, implement and evaluate care in this systematic way. It does not, however, tell nurses *what* to assess or *how* to assess. Nor does nursing process tell us what to include in our care plan or how to set goals and evaluate. The *what* and *how* of care planning can be supplied by a nursing model. Arguments have been put forward by some nurses that one of the reasons for the apparent failure of the nursing process is that we implemented it without a framework to hang it on, namely the framework of a nursing model.

A nursing model is an explanation of the relationship between a person, his/her environment, health, illness and nursing care. Since there are many ways of explaining this relationship, so too are there many models of nursing. It is certainly not a question of which model is right; it is more a question of which model explains the relationship between those concepts in a way which most appropriately matches the nurse's own value system and the needs of the client or client group. In any event, the model chosen becomes the framework on which to carry out the process of nursing. To those who have used different nursing models it soon becomes very clear that assessment of a patient using the Roper, Logan and Tierney model provides different assessment information from an assessment of a patient using the Roy Adaptation model. Part of nursing judgement is choosing the most appropriate model for assessing patients and for planning and evaluating care.

The nursing process and the concept of caring

Recent nursing literature (Benner and Wrubel, 1989; Leininger, 1981; Roach, 1984; Watson, 1979) highlights the concept of caring as the central concept of nursing. Like the nursing process, caring is not just something nurses do. Rather, it is something nurses are. It is a way of being. However, each nurse or group of nurses may have varying definitions of what caring means. This raises a number of questions:

1. What does caring mean for me?
2. Who decides (and how) what is to count as caring?
3. How is caring measured? or indeed, can it be measured?
4. How do different value systems determine what is to count as caring?

One thing is inevitable. In rethinking the nursing process as described throughout this chapter, it is inevitable that it will cause a rethinking of the concept of caring. (*see* Chapters 1 and 8).

Caring can be viewed from a variety of perspectives. The word 'caring' can be defined as in the phrase, 'to take care of.' The notion of caring from this perspective is one of paternalism, or doing something for someone which implies a power relationship or a position of control. Indeed, many of our patients do require nurses to 'take care of them.' Problems arise, however, when the nurse's notion of caring in any nurse-patient situation results in the nurse behaving within a role where she always 'takes care of' her patients. This definition of caring is incongruent with the notion of partnership between nurse and patient as described earlier in this chapter.

An alternative definition of caring is portrayed in the phrase, 'to care for.' To care for someone is subtly different from taking care of someone. Caring for another implies a certain involvement, although perhaps a sympathetic involvement, through the giving of self to the person who is being cared for. However, 'caring for' another can still imply a power relationship of nurse to patient.

A third definition of caring can be described in the phrase, 'to care about' another. Caring *about* someone implies a deeper personal relationship which is about feeling *with* another person, rather than feeling *for* another. Caring about also implies an unconditional type of caring which works within a framework of feeling for the patient's needs rather than the nurses' wishes. In a re-defined process of nursing as described within this chapter, this third definition of caring is the definition which underpins the process of nursing.

Summary

The nursing profession in the United Kingdom began to examine the notion of the process of nursing nearly 15 years ago. However, its limited success and the misunderstanding generated in that time makes it necessary to rethink the nursing process.

To take a fresh look at the nursing process requires a fundamental paradigm shift; a shift from viewing nursing (and nursing process) as tasks, to creating a vision of nursing as a way of thinking, doing and being; a shift from taking control over patients (taking care of patients) to one of partnership (caring about patients); a shift from reacting (doing) to proacting (thinking, doing and being).

This chapter has attempted to offer new explanations of the nursing process within a different paradigm from traditional nursing. Nursing process, as described here, offers a framework for nursing practice which invites the nurse to redefine caring to mean caring *about* people, as opposed to taking care of and caring for people, and to use self as a powerful tool in nursing.

In our new definition of the nursing process, the traditional four stages of nursing process are replaced by a number of activities which together are designed to put into practice a value system based on the principle of respecting the individuality of patients. The activities in the new definition of nursing process include:

- forming and building relationships
- through this relationship, sharing information, thoughts, feelings and noticing non-verbal messages
- reflecting on information gained through the relationship with the patient
- checking out information and perceptions with the patient
- making connections between different pieces of information and drawing some conclusions (nursing diagnosis)
- making tentative decisions about patient needs for nursing, and priorities
- checking these out with the patient to see if he shares these priorities
- setting shared goals or expected outcomes in measurable terms and with evaluation dates
- identifying nursing options with reference to available research, theory or empirical evidence
- choosing particular nursing options and justifying the choice of nursing care prescriptions
- formal monitoring of patient progress with the patient at periodic intervals
- formal evaluation of care against goals or expected outcomes

- changing nursing prescriptions, if necessary, in light of evaluative information.

All the above offer a set of guidelines for thinking and doing; but to make them real requires the 'being' part of nursing, e.g. via the therapeutic use of self. Although 'Therapeutic use of Self' has its origins in psychotherapy (Ersser, 1991) this concept has influenced a number of nurse therapists. Travelbee (1971) wrote that therapeutic use of self requires the educated heart and the educated mind to work together. This implies that therapeutic use of self is about intentional actions on the part of the nurse to promote courage, inner security and self-confidence in the patient (Taylor, 1982).

Travelbee defines 'Therapeutic use of Self' as follows:

> 'When a nurse uses self therapeutically she consciously makes use of her personality and knowledge in order to effect a change in the ill person. This change is considered therapeutic when it alleviates the individual's stress.'

Through the therapeutic use of self in person-to-person partnership with patients the values underpinning individualised, humanistic care make nursing process an intensely human activity, in harmony with the activities of thinking, doing and making professional judgements.

References

Agan, R. D. (1987). Intuitive knowing as a dimension of nursing. *Advances in Nursing Science*, **10(1)**, 63–70.

Aggleton, P. and Chalmers, H. (1986). *Nursing Models and the Nursing Process*. Macmillan, Basingstoke.

Benner, P. and Wrubel, J. (1989). *The Primacy of Caring*. Addison Wesley, Manlo Park.

Donabedian, A. (1969). Quality of Care: problems of measurement 2. Some issues in evaluating the quality of nursing care. *American Journal of Public Health*, **59(10)**, 1833–6.

Ersser, S. (1991). A Search for the Therapeutic dimensions of nurse-patient interactions. In *Nursing as Therapy*, (McMahon and Pearson, Eds). Chapman and Hall, London.

George, J. (Ed.) (1985). *Nursing Theories*. 2nd edn. Prentice-Hall, Englewood Cliffs.

Hunt, J. M. and Marks-Maran, D. (1986). *Nursing Care Plans: the Nursing Process at Work*. 2nd edn. Wiley, Chichester.

Leininger, M. M. (1981). *Caring: an Essential Human Need*. Slack, Thorofare.

Marks-Maran, D. J. (1988). *Skills for Care Planning*. Scutari, London.
Roach, S. (1984). *Caring: the Human Mode of Being – Perspectives in Caring*. University of Toronto, Faculty of Nursing, Toronto.
Taylor, C. (1982). *Mereness' Essentials of Psychiatric Nursing* 11th edn. C. V. Mosby, St Louis.
Travelbee, J. (1971). *Interpersonal Aspects of Nursing* 2nd edn. F. A. Davis, Philadelphia.
United Kingdom Central Council for Nursing, Midwifery and Health Visiting. (1984). *Code of Professional Conduct for the Nurse, Midwife and Health Visitor*. 2nd edn. UKCC, London.
United Kingdom Central Council for Nursing, Midwifery and Health Visiting. (1986). *Project 2000: a New Preparation for Practice*. UKCC, London.
Watson, J. (1979). *Nursing: the Philosophy and Science of Caring*. Little, Brown, Boston.
Yura, H. and Walsh, M. (1983). *The Nursing Process: Assessing, Planning, Implementing, Evaluation*. 4th edn. Appleton-Century-Crofts, Norwalk.

Suggested further reading

Chinn, P. (1985). Debunking myths in nursing theory and research. *Image*, **17** (2) Spring, 45–9.
Field, P. A. (1987). The impact of nursing theory on the clinical decision-making process. *Journal of Advanced Nursing*, **12** (5) Sept, 563–71.
Hurst, K. and Dean, A. (1987). An investigation into nurses' perceptions of problem-solving in clinical practice. In Hannah K. J. *et. al.*, (Eds), pp. 409–11. *Clinical Judgement and Decision-Making: the Future With Nursing Diagnosis*. John Wiley & Sons, New York.
Kobert, L. and Folan, M. (1990). Coming of age in nursing: rethinking the philosophies behind holism and nursing process. *Nursing and Health Care* (6) June, **11**, 308–12.
Robinson, D. (1990). Two decades of 'The Process'. *Senior Nurse*, **10** (2) June, 4–6.
Woolley, N. (1990). Nursing diagnosis: exploring the factors which may influence the reasoning process. *Journal of Advanced Nursing*, **15** (1) Jan, 110–17.

5 Nursing models

The self image of the nurse

The most important gift a nurse can bring to the nurse-patient relationship is herself. The very ability as a nurse, with all the many variables of practice, is more important than wards, beds, equipment or drugs. It is the care-giving process, and is explored fully in the many texts on Primary Nursing (Manthey, 1980; Pearson, 1988; Wright, 1990b).

Nurses who give of self when giving care have to first of all value themselves and value nursing. They need to feel self-confident, comfortable with themselves and assured that what they are offering is valuable and valued. In other words they need to feel happy with their self-perception or self image. Every nurse has a different self-image which is formed through relationships and experience with others. This not only reinforces one's own self-image but also changes it as the reaction of others is experienced. If nurses are confident of their presentation of self, they will react with others naturally, within the role rather than playing at it. They will give of themselves comfortably, and patients will be assured by their presence and actions.

Nurses' self-image is shaped not only by their personal experiences, but by their education as a nurse, their work experiences and their social life. Female nurses' self-image is coloured by the traditional female role in society; that of male nurses by their upbringing which places male role expectations (the provider within the family for example) upon them.

When using a model of nursing the nurse reflects her role defined within the model. How well this is internalised into self-image will depend on how congruent the model is to their individual perception of nursing. A skilled nurse may incorporate the values of several different models within the practice framework, whilst a less skilled nurse may have difficulty in feeling comfortable with one.

The therapeutic use of self, possible only when one is comfortable with one's self-image, is essential to any nurse/patient relationship. 'A pre-requisite for the therapeutic use of self is self-awareness on behalf of the nurse', (Thibodeau, 1983). For positive therapeutic care to ensue the nurse needs a positive valuing of self – a good self-image. To give of self whilst using a model of nursing is essential. Just what one gives is developed in several ways. Firstly the nurse's own self-image and self confidence comes through. This is created, as we have seen, not only by the attitudes, beliefs and ethical values that she has internalised through both her personal and professional development, but also by how others see her. Secondly the nursing theorist also defines the nurse's role within the model application. Finally the environment within which care is given will influence the way the nurse works. Thus an American nurse will practise differently from one within the United Kingdom and a hospital nurse differently from a health visitor, even though all are using the same model.

The uniqueness of the nurse is individual and this develops rather than inhibits, the application of the nursing model. This chapter can offer only one individual's interpretation of the development of self-image in a practitioner; the development of self is so much a personal thing, which the individual nurse must explore through day-to-day practice. This chapter can only aim to offer an understanding of the theorist's perception. However, it should assist the nurse to choose a model which suits the philosophical framework for practice which fits closest to her internalised self-image.

Core components

All nursing models recognise the core components of man – environment, health, and nursing.

The concept of man as the key individual is similar in all nursing models. Sometimes man is seen purely as a physical being (Nightingale, 1859), but many accept that 'the whole is greater than the sum of the parts', exploring issues of psychological and social well-being alongside those of physiological health. Inherent in this image of healthy man is the need for the nurses' self-image to reflect a healthy lifestyle. Many older nurses who trained in the 1950s and 1960s will remember well the control Matrons exhibited in attempts to perpetuate the professional self-image.

Student nurses, and many trained staff, 'lived in', eating in hospital dining rooms where 'healthy' meals were supervised by Matron or her deputy. Nurses 'signed in' after an evening out, ensuring enough sleep (essential for psychological well-being), and social life was disrupted by regulations. Suffice to say, this produced, not unexpectedly, a nurse who was out-of-touch with the realities of the lifestyle which patients and families enjoyed, and one whose idea of health was far removed from that experienced by the many ordinary people for whom she cared.

Increasingly, the public has become aware of the need for the individual to adopt a healthy body-image and is recognising that the way man lives affects his or her health. Politicians in 1991 produced manifestoes which emphasised their responsibility in enabling the individual to live a healthy lifestyle. The role of the nurse, within all nursing models, is to reinforce man as an individual, but, above all, as an individual achieving maximum health potential.

Smoking has long been recognised as a cause of ill-health in the individual; more recently the effects of diet are being acknowledged along with those of alcohol and drug abuse. There is no doubt that the misuse by man of his or her own body causes disease and malfunction. The image of the nurse must therefore be that of a healthy individual. To that end nurses reflect their responsibility to encourage a healthy lifestyle in patients by not smoking in front of them, by trying to maintain weight at an acceptable level, and by not misusing drugs or alcohol.

Florence Nightingale laid great store by a nurse who looked professional. More modern 'Matrons' may interpret her advice in a more relaxed way, expecting nurses at all times to dress *appropriately* for their work environment. The nurses' self-image and self-perception is important if her confidence in care giving is to be obvious to all. A nurse unhappy with her physical appearance cannot educate others into a more acceptable way of life; neither can a nurse who brings psychological or social distress into work be as relaxed and free to care as one would wish. To this end the age of the directive Matron, controlling all aspects of the nurse's life, has gone. Sadly we still have many managers who fail to provide counselling facilities for those who need psychological help to maintain mental health, and who do not recognise their staffs' need for an adequate and relaxing social life. Nurses should try hard to project a self-image of individual health and well-being if they wish to provide a confident role model for patients and families.

The environment in which one lives and works also affects health. Nightingale saw nurses as controlling it, Neuman sees us as manipulating it, Roy as encouraging and assisting patients to adapt to it, and Orem as facilitating care so that patients can live a healthy life within it. Basic assumptions perhaps, but none-the-less effective as a starting point for demonstrating how important a knowledge of, and insight into, the patients environment is for the nurse planning care and carrying out the care plan. This knowledge, of course, brings stress.

Increasingly in the cost effective/efficient environment of the 1990s nurses are identifying needs which cannot be readily met. The stroke patient who needs minor alterations to her home to enable her to return there may find that there is no Local Authority help with meeting the cost. Similarly, the family who lives in a damp house may have to wait many months for re-housing despite the fact their young child has chronic bronchitis. It has become increasingly difficult for families on Income Support to manage to meet day-to-day living expenses. Houses are cold, diet is poor, and the result is ill-health. The nurse needs empathy for those patients caught in this cycle of deprivation since only by recognising its existence and helping patients and family challenge it, can they move through it into a more healthy lifestyle.

Health as the key to all care and treatment actions is a common theme in all nursing models. It has moved from merely 'an absence of disease' into:

> '"completeness" or "wholeness" of mind and body.'
>
> (Henderson, 1966)

> 'the complete state of physical, psychological and social well-being.'
>
> (World Health Organization, 1946)

> '" a state of wellness" or "optimal functioning".'
>
> (Riehl-Sisca, 1989)

> 'wellness is the ability to maintain equilibrium.'
>
> (Neuman, 1982)

> 'a state of integration and wholeness.'
>
> (Roy, 1984)

A nurse with a positive self-image will reflect a healthy lifestyle, look healthy, and reflect a state of wellness. In exploring the concept of health and wellness it is important to recognise that, by 1989, the profession's theorists were defining health as optimal functioning, not total wellness. Thus a person who is physically or mentally disabled can still be defined as healthy. The impact of this on the patient's self-image must not be undervalued. It has led directly to the disappearance of the labelling (or stigmatisation) of some patients as 'chronic-sick' and has introduced such concepts as active rehabilitation programmes for patients with cancer or other life-threatening diseases. We now accept that those with diabetes or epilepsy can be well; indeed many models (e.g. Roy) actively encourage nurses to help patients and families make the necessary adaptive changes to reach their maximum health potential.

Health is increasingly seen as a state of total equilibrium, both of body and mind and nurses are becoming much more aware of the needs of patients and families as these relate to social and psychological health. Thus we link back into the core element of the patient's environment and are required to explore the links which this has with health – the total health of the individual.

Nursing. In reading about nursing models one quickly perceives that each model uses nursing differently, and when using different models the nurse needs to adopt a different role. For example Wright (1990a) defines the nurse as a healer, using therapeutic skills. He gives the key functions as support, rehabilitation, help (especially mentioning helping patients to die with dignity) and innovation. Neuman (1982) explores the concepts of care-giving, communication, teaching and co-ordinating, whilst Parse (1981) focuses on 'human-to-human inter-relationships' within 'a caring, healing perspective'.

Whilst each theorist has commonalities, there are obvious differences in the way nursing is perceived and therefore the role, and thus the self-image that is assumed. Perhaps the only central theme in all the theories is that of intervention; the nurse as an active participant working with the patient (and, when appropriate, family and friends) to achieve openly acknowledged and stated goals. The uniqueness comes from the way the nurse 'intervenes'. Aggleton and Chalmers (1986) delineate different roles to those of Wright, Neuman and Parse, which are perhaps more encompassing. They use such terms as 'physician's assistant', 'patients advocate', 'constant presence', 'facilitator of self-care' and 'modifier of behavioural patterns'. Nurses will recognise that they are all of these at different times and in different places.

The nurse as a healer

For almost a century nurses in the United Kingdom followed the task allocation approach to care described by Nightingale. Patients had things done to them, treatments and isolated tasks performed upon them and these were delivered within a routine of ward orders and lists. The age-old therapeutic skills of massage, relaxation, and hypnosis had been moved sideways, or indeed lost altogether, as the profession moved (as did the doctors) into a world where anything that could be prescribed (tablets, treatments, care) was seen as 'good', and anything that did not involve routine and structure was 'inappropriate'.

Nurses are moving towards recognising that positive nursing intervention can reduce, and even occasionally eliminate, the need for drugs and invasive treatment. Recognising that a patient who is relaxed heals quicker, be it in mind or body, the nurse who practises therapeutic nursing will first aim to assist this relaxation. In the beginning this will be accomplished by listening to the patient; letting him talk out his anxieties in a quiet place, answering questions, explaining options and, above all, expressing interest and concern, thus helping the relaxation process.

Nurses too are developing skills in massage, aiding relaxation and pain control by using the traditional skills of a masseuse, accompanied by appropriate oils and creams (aromatherapy). By using essential oils appropriately, a gradual and long-lasting relaxation can be achieved. Oils can be used in burners, to create a conducive environment, as well as for massage, and in inhalations. A list of oils, and their uses, is given in Table 5.1 at the end of this chapter.

As with all therapeutic nursing skills, the practitioner must be sure that he or she has received proper instruction by a registered practitioner. The National Boards for Nursing, Midwifery and Health Visiting are beginning to approve courses which have massage and aromatherapy as component modules, and there are several private centres which offer courses taught by Registered Practitioners.

Increasingly, nurses are also developing skills as counsellors. Skilled counsellors are able not only to assess the complex emotional problems patients and families face, but are able to help the patients review the options and often resolve the dilemma. Counselling also requires expertise, and all nurses should ensure they are taught to not only counsel patients at an appropriate level, but also to recognise when a skilled therapist should be consulted. Counselling is commonly one area where the nurse needs to remember 'fools rush in where angels fear to tread'.

Chiropractice or chirotherapy is another area where nurses are developing skills. Chirotherapists treat muscle and joint-related problems using manipulation of joints and the spinal column. It may be used alongside the manipulation of muscles (massage) or by itself. The primary aim of the manipulation is to reduce pressure, and initial diagnosis is made by touch and pressure prodding over the areas about which the patient complains.

Some nurses are developing skills in acupuncture, having been taught by therapists who have studied this historical Eastern approach to pain relief and relaxation. Others recommend reflexology, which is based on similar principles of referred pressure, or the more modern TENS (Trans-Electrical Nerve Stimulation).

Unlike much drug therapy, many of these interventions can result in total body well-being. The nurse wishing to learn more about therapeutic practice can contact: The Council for Complementary and Alternative Medicine, Suite 1, 19a Cavendish Square, London, W1M OAD.

Nurses who work as healers, practising therapeutic skills, often find a great personal satisfaction. These skills can be used alongside and in support of conventional treatment (in conditions such as AIDS, and Cancer), or may prove successful in their own right. This is more often true with chronic disorders, such as allergies, sciatica, or in assisting patients over acute incidents (sprains, and torn ligaments). Using these skills helps nurses develop the 'human-to-human inter-relationships' (Parse 1981) needed for all successful care-giving. Many skills can also be taught to patients and families, so that such intervention can continue at home.

Core elements

The core elements can thus be seen as common to all models, becoming specific in the way they are interpreted, applied, or developed. But whichever way the nurse chooses to practise model-based care there is no doubt that her perception of nursing care, and the way she practises, will ensure the model is interpreted almost always in a way that is unique.

But although core elements are common, the models themselves do differ, and in order for the nurse to project a comfortable self-image she needs to ensure she chooses one which suits her own perceptions of nursing and which enables her to practise as she would wish.

Nightingale (1859)

It is not the purpose of this chapter to argue whether or not Florence Nightingale was a theorist and thus her work a model. Suffice to say that within Nightingale's work the nurse will recognise the common components of a nursing model and will note that the role of the nurse is clearly defined. The role of 'lady probationer' produced a very clear self-image. The nurse was a doctor's assistant, a controller and manipulator of the environment, as well as being a teacher, and an organiser. Nightingale's writings stress the need for management, direction of others, teaching of both patient and family and 'strict discipline'. Many older nurses will remember Matrons who trained under this model – one was always sure of their self-image! However, Nightingale also stressed the need to listen carefully to patients and families before making decisions (perhaps the first recognition of a nursing assessment) and the role of the nurse as a patient's advocate.

The medical model of care

Nightingale's model led nursing directly into the medical model. Her definition of the nurse as the doctor's assistant took priority over all else. The self-image is clearly defined as subservience to the doctor. It has taken over a century for nurses to rise above this self-image, and indeed others' perception of them in this role; but there is no doubt that the image portrayed by Hattie Jacques in the 'Carry On' films personified the handmaiden role.

However, the medical model was more than this and led to a self-image which still persists today. The nurse working with a medical model has been accused of two alternatives, but not necessarily conflicting, approaches to care. First the image of efficiency, carrying out tasks of care, in a skilled, and professional way. Check lists and workbooks proliferated. The whole framework was marked by order and structure, not least so in the presentation of the nurse herself; always female, always a hospital nurse, always in starched uniform, and always capable and confident. This image has largely become historical, as more men join the profession and as nurses move into community care and out of uniform. This emphasises the nurse as an independent practitioner and an individual accepting personal accountability. The public perception mirrors the confident self-image thus portrayed.

However, the Nightingale model has bequeathed another legacy, that of extended role; that of doctor's assistant for the 1990s. December 1990 saw the release of the advance letter from the Department of Health (1990) on Junior Doctors' Hours. In the letter the Department of Health recognises the role of the nurse in taking on junior doctors' tasks. Care will be needed if the nurse is not to become the doctor's assistant all over again. One goal for the 1990s will be to ensure that the development of the extended role is achieved within a nursing context; within the framework of nursing practice, presenting the image of the nurse as an independent practitioner, an autonomous decision maker and not a scavenger, picking up the work doctors don't want. If this were to happen the nurse would be retracing steps back to a pure Nightingale model, which would be a truly retrograde move.

For three or four decades now nursing has been moving forwards towards independent, autonomous practice. As nurses become better skilled and better educated their self-image and their professional image improve. Independent practice is about being a member, an equal member, of the health care team. It is this equality that will ensure the nurse's self-image in the 21st Century and which will differ from that of the 20th.

Henderson (1966)

Virginia Henderson's work is perhaps the watershed, the Rubicon between the past and the future. Henderson recognised the nurse as an equal member of the health care team, the 'initiator and controller' of her own nursing actions. But she modifies this interpretation by her recognition or acceptance that the nursing care plan is carried out within the therapeutic medical plan. Thus she presents the nurse with a confused image, a less than clearly defined role.

Henderson did however, clearly recognise the need for the nurse to work with the patient in a non-directive capacity ' . . . assisting the patient, sick or well, in the performance of those activities . . . ' Henderson saw the nurse as the intelligent helper, interpreting the needs of the patient and family, correlating these with the medical treatment plan and agreeing a nursing care plan which enables patient, family, friends, nurse, and doctor, as a care team, to achieve the defined self care goals. Wright (1990a) identifies helping concepts as basic, integral and essential to nursing practice and clearly acknowl-edges the debts the modern professional nurse owes to Nightingale and Henderson.

Henderson was also the first nurse author to acknowledge the complexity of nursing, which becomes apparent when nurses move away from the Nightingale, medical model, and the task-orientated practice modes of the 1950s and 1960s. The place of nursing as a therapy is defined clearly in her work, and she places special emphasis on the role of the nurse in caring for the terminally ill. When giving care to those patients the cool, calm, peaceful image of the nurse is paramount. Later in her work she explores the nurse's role in other areas of care. When caring for a newborn baby e.g., the image she must present to the family is that of 'knowledgeable doer', even though this may not be the perception she has of herself. When working in the intensive care unit, the nurse must project alertness, efficiency, and specialist skill; a perception every nurse tries hard to internalise and make explicit.

Finally, Henderson has much to say about the nurse as a teacher, recognising that the skilled teacher passes knowledge and expertise on to others through her presentation of self as a confident practitioner.

As with any nursing act, the nurse working with Henderson's model needs to project self-confidence and assurance; qualities which only come when she, herself, is valued.

Human-needs model

Using a human-needs model such as Henderson's places many respon-sibilities on the nurse. She must develop high level communication skills, probably becoming a non-directive counsellor who brings nurs-ing knowledge to expert levels, assisting the patient to make appropri-ate health care choices which ensure deficits in human needs are met.

The human-needs model demands considerable nurse-patient trust in that the patient needs to expose weaknesses, anxieties, social deficits, problems and family stresses to the nurse so that assistance can be provided and support given. The nurse also has to be able to encourage patients, families, and friends to discuss psychological problems, some of which, in being verbalised, are being brought to the surface for the first time. The nurse therefore in using a human needs model must be comfortable as a confidante and as a counsellor.

Other Human-Needs Models which are used to-day in the United Kingdom include the works of Roper, Logan and Tierney (1985) and Minshull *et. al.* (1986). Roper, Logan and Tierney see nurses as 'the link between complicated, technical medical care and the maintenance of everyday bodily and mental functions which are so critical to the patient's comfort and so important to him as a person'. Minshull *et. al.*, also discuss support, with the nurse helping the patient meet those needs that cannot be met alone. All therefore make the same or similar demands on the nurse, namely the expectation of an insightful, supportive counsellor. The weaknesses in the models lie not in the nurse's self-perception, nor how the model is applied in practice, but in the very approach.

In the present socio-economic and political climate (1991) health care needs are frequently identified (and from the medical perspective treatment demands) which cannot be met. The conflict of frustration and despair this produces in patient and nurse (and also the doctor, or indeed within the health-care team) can traumatise what should be a therapeutic and therefore constructive relationship.

The nurse therefore needs to become politically aware, recognising the constraints which can traumatise the nurse-patient relationship. When the relationship is affected by, for example, the nurse's inability to meet a newly identified need, the value of nursing diminishes in the eyes of the patient, and the nurse feels bad about her quality of care. Thus her perception of self changes. Nurses become frustrated by being inhibited from giving the quality of care they wish, and it may be that we need to move to explore alternatives which are more cost-effective than those we have turned to in the past.

Pearson (1988) and Wright (1990b) both explore the cost-effectiveness of active therapeutic nursing where nurse and patient work in a one-to-one relationship. Thus 'primary' nursing relies on this relationship to build up trust, and patients and their families need to actively participate in meeting the goals set by the care planning process. Within such a relationship the nurse feels valued.

It could be easier to use a human-needs model within the framework of individualised patient care, since the depth of trust may allow alternatives of care and treatment to be explored, and also allow the nurse to admit that there is no easy solution, perhaps no solution at all! It may, indeed, be the only way to maintain the therapeutic relationship through the conflict and despair which occurs when identified needs cannot be met.

Systems models

The best known systems models are American, but have been used with some success in this country. Neuman (1982) and Roy (1984) present adaptation models using nursing intervention to achieve change within the patient's social, psychological and physical environment.

Neuman describes the levels of nursing intervention as: primary/ preventative; secondary/acute response; tertiary/ rehabilitative. She sees the nurse's role as assisting the patient to make the adaptive changes necessary to stabilise body systems. Thus the role is one of change-agent and the nurses self-image must recognise leadership arising from a wide-ranging knowledge base which provides insight into the changes needed.

Neuman identifies two lines of defence which protect the patient from stress or stressors. These the patient uses constructively to achieve necessary adaptation. It must be remembered though that the patient may also use these lines of defence to 'maladapt' or to make inappropriate changes. The flexible line is seen as dynamic, mainly concerned with short-term adaptive behaviours, and the nurse must assume the role of guide or facilitator. Thus the patient having general anaesthesia and a reduction in fluid intake will have the usual defence line against dehydration (physiological thirst triggers) inhibited by the 'nil orally' requirement. The nurse has to first of all ensure that the patient, and any visitors, psychologically adapt to being thirsty by explaining the reasons for the inhibition. The physiological need for homeostatic balance will be met by an alternative defence line, such as an intravenous infusion. The flexibility of the dynamic adaptation ensures that the homeostatic integrity of the individual is maintained.

The change-agent role of the nurse is practised at a more highly skilled level when permanent adaptation is the order of the day. Thus adaptation may be primarily physiological, such as dietary change, but the skilled nurse will recognise and plan care to achieve the social, psychological and environmental adaptation needed as well. The nurse may need to enlist the support of family, friends, work or classmates as the adaptation goals are achieved.

Roy's model also places the nurse in the role of change-agent demanding the confident self-image inherent in the change process mechanism. She recognises man as having four sub-systems: physiological, self-concept or self perception, role and interdependency. The nurse must work alongside the patient to assist in the achievement of adaptation changes within these systems. This will maintain and/or improve health. The nurse's knowledge base facilitates appropriate decision-making and her self-presentation to the patient is that of the key worker in the change process necessary to facilitate acceptance of the essential adaptation process.

In order to work as a change-agent one needs first to understand the process of change. Berman and McLaughlin (1976) recognise a 3-stage process for educational change, and nursing practice innovation can surely be recognised as educational change, which they describe as initiation, implementation and incorporation.

Initiation phase. This defines the processes which lead up to the need for change being identified, and ends as the decision is made to implement it. The nurse assessing the patient would identify a need for change, and would complete the initiation phase by discussing the plan with the patient and family and (hopefully) agreeing how and when to move forward with it. Using the Neuman model the nurse will identify the stressors and negotiate with the patient (if appropriate) the way adaptation will be achieved.

Implementation. This is recognised as the care giving phase, actively involving the patient in understanding the care process as far as possible, and ensuring the reasons for decisions made are clearly understood. Only then can the patient work constructively to achieve adaptation.

Incorporation. This occurs when the change is internalised and (using Neuman) adaptation is complete and homeostasis is achieved. As with all change processes the stages intermingle and interlink. In using care planning the plan may be in a more advanced stage with one goal than with another. The skilled practitioner will recognise this and use her knowledge of the change process to work with the patient and family through whichever model is the chosen base for practice.

Development models

These are less familiar to British nurses and little is written demonstrating their use here. This is possibly because they address nursing as an emerging science discipline, whether social-scientific, bio-physical or existentialist in approach. They include the works of Rogers (1979), Parse (1981), Watson (1979) and Riehl-Sisca (1989). The nurse using these models must employ scientific principles to guide delivery of care. The self-concept internalised must therefore be that of a practitioner comfortable with the scientific framework who can function as a change-agent within the remit of the various models.

Other models

One of the non-nursing theorists who has influenced nursing practice in nurse teaching over the last thirty years is Abraham Maslow (1970). Minshull's work is based on Maslow, and can be included as one of the human needs models. He views people from a perspective based on human value and human worth. Maintaining self-care at an appropriate level is the individual's responsibility. Nursing intervention is necessary when these self-care needs cannot be met alone. The nurse must endeavour to encourage self-esteem and self-value in patients, and must demonstrate these qualities to them.

Campbell (1984) is a theological philosopher, whose work crosses from nursing into other disciplines and can therefore be seen as a framework for multi-disciplinary care. He defined professional care as 'moderated love which combines necessary detachment with a concern for individual values and socio-political change'. This he refers to as 'skilled companionship', where the nurse walks with the patient, family and friends through a journey centred on partnership in care, and the journey ending only when adaptation is achieved or a peaceful death ensues. Exploring Campbell's philosophical approach leads one to suggest that it allows us to deliver care within the most natural of self-concepts, that of friend and companion; the most natural of roles, and the one most people are comfortable with. However, many nurses are still uncomfortable with the 'closeness' model-based practice and, the nursing process brings. Some find it threatening, others worry about the accountability placed on them, whilst others question their knowledge and ability to understand what are still seen as new approaches to care. It may be that Campbell's ideas are more congruent with the self-image that the 1990s may bring.

Conclusion

Overall, nurses working with models need self-confidence. This will only come when the nurse is comfortable with the necessary knowledge base, personal responsibility and accountability, and has freedom to choose which model is most appropriate for which patient. Once the nurse is confident of her role, her self-concept will grow to match it.

We are moving in this direction – the second goal for the 1990s must be to ensure we achieve it.

The role of the patient

'In most hospitals the patient cannot eat as he wishes; his freedom of movement is curtailed; his privacy invaded; he is put in bed in strange nightclothes that make him feel as unattractive as a punished child; he is separated from the objects of his affection; he is deprived of almost every diversion of his normal day; deprived of work and often reduced to dependence on persons who often are younger than he is, and sometimes less intelligent and courteous.'

(Henderson, 1966)

In her book, Henderson describes a not unfamiliar picture of the role of the patient at a time when nurses practised task allocation and supported the medical model of care. A similar description is found in

Goffman's (1961) 'Asylums.' Both authors describe patients as people placed in a dependent role, having things done to them, 'freed' from decision making, having no say in what happens to them, no choice and no individuality. Whereas Henderson likens this picture to a child's role, Goffman equates it with the image of a prisoner or a resident of a closed psychiatric unit. Although the references are now old, the situation can occasionally be recognised in some of the long-stay units today.

Choice is something we all value, and are encouraged to exercise from our earliest days. Young infants are positively motivated towards choosing toys or stories; later toddlers select T-shirts and socks, moving on to choosing drinks, then an ice-cream or ice-lolly, and their outfit for the day. As they come to school-age, the rejection of uniform, and the later (teenage) adoption of trends in dress and behaviour all reflect society's desire to allow individuals to make choices.

As adults we criticise those who can't decide between tea or coffee, or who 'fence sit' when called upon to be decisive. Choice is part of our lifestyle, yet for so long nurses and doctors have removed any decision making away from patients. This applies to such simple decisions as, for example to dress or not to dress, to eat or not to eat, through to failing to provide patients with sufficient information about their condition and possible treatment options and outcomes. This latter ensures they cannot make an informed choice.

Just as the protection British medical staff enjoy allows them to justify not offering the treatment choices, many nurses still see institutionalisation as the reason for not offering even simple choices. Does it really make a difference whether patients dress or don't dress whilst in Investigation Units? Why can't they go to the hospital dining room where choice of food is available? Anyone who has spent time in Scandinavian, Dutch or German hospitals will appreciate the choice patients there enjoy.

Nursing models are about choice; the nurse's right to select a model which allows her to care for a patient in the way she wishes and to consult with the patient about how that care is given. Johnson's model (1980) recognises that people have choices to make in life, and that these choices are affected by not only new information but by their socialisation and experience. A choice previously made which had a favourable outcome is much more likely to be made a second time than is a choice which resulted in distress or disagreement. Thus the wise nurse ascertains the patient's life experiences and uses that knowledge to assist the patient to exercise choices in health care options. Johnson supports the nurse's need to advise on choices but recognises the right of the individual concerned to have the final say. The definition of individual is, for Johnson, always the patient. I can find no reference to parent-role, 'significant other' role or family decision making.

However this issue is confused, especially where nurses' ethics are concerned, and there are frequent instances reported in the national press which recognise the confusion between adolescents, and those with mental health problems who wish to make different choices from those decisions guardians may make for them. The nurse must always acknowledge that the primary role she has to facilitate for her patient is that of ensuring he or she is an individual. This is not to say the nurse has to support the patient's choice, but she does have an obligation to ensure the patient's voice is heard.

Role

Patients, like nurses, have many roles. One may ask the question, 'what is a role'?

> 'All the world's a stage,
> And all the men and women merely players;
> They have their exits and their entrances;
> And one man in his time plays many parts . . . '
> (Shakespeare *As you like it*, Act II, Scene VII)

Role theory recognises that individuals have many roles, complexly linking and interlinking one with another. Some are open (or overt), whilst others we keep closed (or covert). We have roles which conflict and others which are comfortably compatible. Role perspective is constantly changing, both because of the individual's own behaviour and because of the implications of outside influences. Any individual exists in an almost constant climate of adaptation necessary to maintain homeostatic equilibrium in all its many and varied perspectives.

The individual

The individual in the centre of the diagram (Fig. 5.1) invariably presents to the nurse as a patient or a client. As we have seen, the primary role we must ascribe to any patient is that of the individual. Elliot-Cannon (1990) defines the terms 'patient' or 'client' as 're-flect(ing) a belief in the recipient of care as a valued person, receiving a service within which they have at least equal rights, and a valued role and status'. All nursing models value the patient; it is the medical models which denigrate people who need care into biological frameworks of anatomy, physiology and disease complexities. Aggleton and Chalmers (1986) define this as 'interrelated sets of anatomical parts and physiological systems'. Whereas the nurse uses knowledge of these subjects to enhance assessments and interaction skills, within a

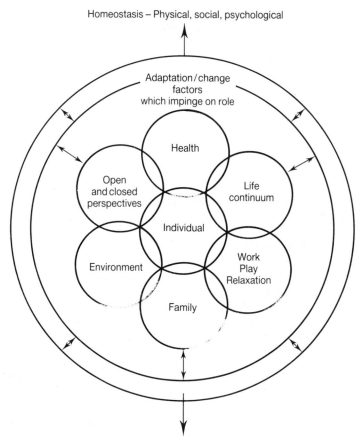

Homeostasis – Physical, social, psychological

Adaptation/change
factors
which impinge on role

Health

Open
and closed
perspectives

Life
continuum

Individual

Environment

Work
Play
Relaxation

Family

Homeostasis, physical, social and psychological

Fig. 5.1

medical model the knowledge base can become an end in itself. The patient role is to be the passive recipient of treatment, accepting advice and direction submissively. Each nursing model though, sees the person/patient as central within the four core elements. It is exactly *how* each theorist sees them that differs. The role of the patient as an individual, a participant, a key decision-maker is common to all models.

Nightingale

Nightingale's model, or philosophical approach, supported the medical model. The patient, and indeed his or her family, fulfilled a passive role within the framework of care. Nightingale focused on the importance of the patient resting within a positively controlled healing environment which was created by the nurse. The patient was the passive recipient of care given by the nurse, and submissively respected the doctor from whom treatment was dispensed. Patients were people to whom things happened, and who had little say in just what exactly was happening.

Nightingale encouraged the nurse to see the patient as someone who must be assisted and supported, within a healthy (by 1860 standards) structured environment which she and the doctor planned, created and enforced. The passive role of the patient was reinforced, as to a certain extent it still is, by the medical staff who maintain a 'mystique' regarding their abilities; and by nurses who support the medical model by task allocation and the accompanying subservient nursing practice.

Henderson (1966)

Virginia Henderson sees the patient as a person with individual needs, whether sick or well. She emphasises the role of the patient as a participant in care planning and the meeting of identified need deficits. The patient, not the doctor or the nurse, appears to have moved to the centre of the role perspective (Fig. 5.1) assuming the key position. In order to enable him to fulfill this key role the nurse provides the knowledge the patient needs; knowledge about the condition, the treatment options and the choices concerning rehabilitation and future life expectancy. This lays the onus on the nurse to fulfill the role as information giver within the care team.

Some patients are anxious about being involved in the decision making process and need encouragement. This is especially true of the older individual whose cultural expectations are that entry into health care means they will be passive recipients, not active participants. However, I believe Henderson casts the patient in the supporting role rather than the star part, since she sees the nurse as the gate-keeper to the information the patient needs to make decisions and then interprets medical treatment and directions. However active a participant the patient wishes to be, the nurse still controls the admission to participation. Whether the doctor or the nurse is the key player in Henderson's model must therefore remain a matter for debate.

Human-needs models

All human needs models see the patient in the role of active participant in care. Orem (1985) sees the goal of nursing as developing the patient's self-care activities/abilities until role function is at its maximum and the patient is the primary provider. She recognises that physical or psychological deficits make some patients (e.g. the amputee or the schizophrenic) unable to develop total role competency but desires the nurse to strive, with the patient, to become as independent and self-sufficient as possible. The role of nurse, patient, family member, and friend interlink to achieve these goals.

For the healthy person, Orem's model requires the individual to accept the responsibility for maintaining health, for accepting health education and for taking an active role in the prevention of infection and disease. This lays the onus on the nurse to 'practise what is preached' in that the healthy individual (the nurse) is a role model for others. Thus the nurse who smokes, even if not in front of patients, must be aware of the negative role model offered to patients by the smell of smoke on uniform etc. In other words, performed role (what one actually does) must portray the positive health care message if patients are going to internalise a healthy life-style from a positive role model.

Roper, Logan and Tierney (1985) recognise the role conflict that arises as patients enter care. They cite the example of a young mother who, on becoming ill, has to accept rather than give care, and that of a managing director who has, for a time, to accept direction rather than direct others. Their book discusses at length the various role perspectives patients have in life and the confusion that arises as they have to adapt to care situations. The goal of the nurse however, is to help the patient to move along the dependence/interdependence continuum from total dependence to maximum independence, assuming the role of self-carer.

Wright (1990a) also recommends the use of a human needs model with the patient actively participating in his or her own care. He develops this further (1990b) in his work on primary nursing where the patient role is not only that of active and equal partner but also holds their own nursing notes and is party to all decision making affecting treatment and care. He sees his model as totally patient-centred, unlike Henderson's, and thus one in which the patient occupies the centre of the role diagram. (*see* Fig. 5.1)

Systems models

The two most widely used systems models in the United Kingdom are those of Neuman (1982) and Roy (1984). Roy recognises that a person adapts according to individual needs which include psychological changes in role when these are necessary. People also change role function as they perceive a need to function differently. The patient works with the nurse to make necessary adaptational changes in role. Thus the role is one of active partnership aiming to achieve independence. However, the patient role is more that of constant change-agent to maintain adaptation (homeostaic balance) rather than achievement (and then a level maintenance) of self-care needs as seen with previous models.

Neuman's model explores stressors which affect the stability of the individual. These stressors can be intra-personal (the person's self-image and self-perception), inter-personal (how he or she relates with those close to them), and extra-personal (how the individual relates to the world at large). All these stressors make demands on the individual and the role he or she plays in the 'game of life'. The patient is assisted towards role stability, and the stabilisation or reduction of the stressors, through active partnership either as an individual or with the group. But, yet again, because the stressors themselves cannot ever be seen as permanently adapted, the patient role is that of self-change agent, constantly adapting role to meet need.

Other models of care

Campbell (1984) whose framework for caring companionship is briefly discussed earlier, casts the patient as an equal partner, jointly responsible with the nurse for the shared journey that is the caring trajectory. It is an interesting perspective and one which leads straight into the Primary Nursing perspective which is perhaps the way forward into the future. Thus model-based practice can be seen as a way to place the patient in the centre of the diagram in the primary role of an individual.

Other roles

Having acknowledged that nursing models clearly place the patient in the centre of the stage it is appropriate to explore other roles which he or she may be required to acknowledge when in a health care setting, be it hospital or community.

Life continuum

The individual's role within the life continuum is one of our roles which is culturally identified. Many countries and cultures, e.g., Mediterranean societies, and those from the Indian sub-continent revere and respect the elderly, giving them a valued role as advisor and counsellor within the community. This is in marked contrast to the Northern European culture where the elderly may be placed in residential care, or are largely neglected by families and societies. Similarly, children and young people in these cultures may expect to have decisions made for them (such as marriage agreements) which Western teenagers would not accept.

Culture too, may be based on previous relationships. We have already acknowledged that older patients, whose introduction to health care when younger was in a framework where others made decisions, may find it difficult to exercise individual choice. Many older patients have an inbred deference to nurses, and find it difficult to respond to the relaxed approach to care that model-based practice can bring. Patients can have difficulty coming to terms with changes forced upon them through the life continuum. The classic example is that of the new mother, whose role conflicts with that of a young wife, and who is torn apart by these conflicting demands. Equally stressful, and known to cause psychological and psychiatric distress, are the changes in role forced upon parents as children become teenagers, demand independence and finally leave home. If these lifestyle changes in role come at the same time as major ill-health, the role stress can inhibit the healing process.

Health

The health of the individual impinges on role. In the previous chapter the definitions of health were explored and we have seen how those with disabilities can maintain a healthy lifestyle and role within society if society will let them. But ill health forces different role conflicts. Increasingly nurses are becoming aware of the role conflict, especially that of sexuality, which results from intervention causing body-image problems. Breast surgery, colostomy formation, or prostatic enlargement are perhaps the immediate and most common examples. More traumatic are those which demand a permanent change in role; the injury which is so severe that the patient cannot contemplate returning to his old job; or the debilitating illness which stops a woman controlling her home. Anxiety about health can affect the way individuals behave, and affect the choices they make. Nurses need to be supportive, to listen non-judgementally, and to be prepared to offer advice. However, one needs to beware of patients choosing options which are quickest (i.e. surgery for breast malignancy over radiotherapy) just because they assume they will be able to return to their usual role more speedily.

Open and closed perspectives

These can be defined as those concepts we acknowledge as affecting our role (i.e. those which are explicit) and those which we do not acknowledge. As an example, consider the young woman who is a practising catholic and who decides not to have an abortion but to carry on with the unplanned pregnancy. Because she makes public her religious objection, her decision to assume the role of unmarried mother is accepted by her society, albeit they may still condemn the sexual activity which caused it. However, the now frankly and publicly agnostic young woman may equally well oppose abortion but is unable to rationalise her decision, failing to remember the influence her Catholic upbringing will have had at the convent school she attended as a child. Similarly, a businessman who, supporting Thatcherism, seeing unemployment as somehow self created, may fail to admit his redundancy even to himself, going out each morning and returning each evening as usual so that his family do not identify his change in role. Issues like this will colour how patients respond and react as individual decision-makers in the health care environment.

Environment

The environment itself of course affects role, socially, culturally and politically. The political framework of today, with its purchaser/provider ethos, places patients into definitive health care settings, thus removing choice from them unless they can afford to pay. Thus a family who wants a natural childbirth, or to use a water-bath, may well have this choice refused. Politics too, affects the community care available, and the social service support which patients need on return after hospitalisation. A nursing model may identify active rehabilitation, the patient may exercise choice and wish to avail himself of this option, but this is all of no substance if the local authority does not employ speech, physio or occupational therapists for the choice to be put into action. Housing also affects health, as does the area in which one lives. How can the respiratory cripple, living in a fourth floor flat without lift access, exercise choice in social activities, aware though he may be of his need to get out and socialise in the fresh air?

Family

We have already seen how family demands, constraints and expectations affect the role of the patient as an individual. This is especially true when the patient is disabled in mind or body. One of the nurse's key tasks may be to assist the family in adapting to 'letting go'; to letting the patient exercise choice. Parents especially have problems in moves into community care for disabled young people or the adolescent with a learning difficulty. Families too, force decisions on to individuals. Refusing treatment or blood transfusions for children is fortunately a rare extreme, but there are instances where parents neglect to bring their children for advised dental treatment, ophthalmic examination or immunisation, thus endangering their health. The nurse needs to assume her advocacy role here, to ensure that her patient has the right to choice.

Work, play and relaxation

These factors obviously affect choice, since most require us to function as part of a team, club, or working group. One's ability to fit back into this group affects individual choice. People put off treatment until after examinations, until a major contract is signed, or until the football game they wish to compete in has been played. With non-acute health interventions this is acceptable; indeed many people pay health insurance just to get this freedom of choice. More serious, and of more concern to the nurse, are those patients under pressure to choose quick options because of outside demands, or the athlete who is pressurised to continue running or playing using drugs when rest and physiotherapy is the obvious essential intervention.

Role balance

Nursing assessment, using the nursing process, based on a nursing model, aims to identify the factors which impinge upon the patient exercising his or her role as an individual. The aim must be to ensure role balance, where compatibility of the multiple roles enables choice to be made and appropriate care and treatment to be given. The aim is obviously total homeostatic balance and the maintenance of optimal health.

The nurse familiar with Campbell's philosophy will find this perception of care congruent. Campbell (1984) defines care as 'moderated love, which combines necessary detachment with a concern for individual values and socio-political change'. The nurse needs to familiarise herself with the local community ethos to ensure she understands the environment and culture within which her patient and family lives, works and plays. Campbell in his work advises on giving care within a relationship that is a partnership rather than the Nightingale concept of the nurse as the manager and the patient as the managed.

The way forward

In May 1991 William Waldegrave, as Secretary of State for Health, announced the award of £3.2 million to develop Nursing Development Units. Within his paper he identified the advantages of primary nursing. Primary nursing empowers patients, strengthens their role within health care settings and encourages them to take a lead role as initiators in their own health care. Primary nursing gives the lead role in 24-h care to the nurse, who, in turn, develops the confidence to allow patients to take the lead role in their own care. The goal of primary nursing must be to make the patient independent.

Ersser and Tutton (1991) define the role of the patient within a primary nursing unit as a true partnership involving 'the adoption of a non-directive style whereby the nurse attempts to give the patient greater choice to help him become a more active participant in his care'. This clearly moves the role of the patient from passive partner, and lays the onus on the nurse to ensure that the patient has all the information needed to make an informed choice. This partnership is more active than those envisaged by Henderson, Orem or Roy. It requires the nurse to ensure the patient functions independently, as far as is possible, from the moment he or she enters care. The individual patient brings into the patient role previous life experiences and knowledge. They bring cultural perceptions, family links, and social class expectations (if class can be recognised as still existing in United Kingdom society of the 1990s).

Some will have extensive knowledge already about their health and treatment needs; some will have very firm ideas about treatment expectations and goals. They may understand why they are in need of nursing care or they may not. Within a primary nursing framework the nurse has to work to ensure the patient has the lead role and is assisted to maintain it.

Summary

All of us have roles which we live with all the time. They reflect our day-to-day activities, within which we (hopefully) can exhibit self-confidence and feel comfortable enough to take on new experiences. New challenges, tackled from a secure role-base, with a comfortable self-image, secure family environment and a circle of friends and colleagues are minimally threatening. The patient role lasts for the minimal time necessary, with adaptive changes taking place in the shortest possible time and with the least disruption.

Nursing comes into its own when the patient lacks a secure role concept, with all that it entails. The patient not only needs to develop a comfortable self-image, but has to be assisted to make lifestyle changes leading to physiological balance and will need help to move into society at large. The medical or surgical help patients need to move into a new role is often physical or arrived at in meeting physical self-care deficits. Where body-image changes, as in amputation or stoma formation, psychological and social role adaptation is necessary. When the patient has learning difficulties or psychiatric disorders, role adaptation may take longer; may indeed need permanent support from the health care team, and will involve primarily both psychological and social adaptation with some physiological support. With many of these patients, as with children, supportive family involvement is essential if the positive role changes are to be effectively achieved.

Whichever approach to care the nurse supports, all modern nursing theorists see the role autonomy of the patient as paramount. The patient has to be assisted to move from role dependency to independence and to maintain independence, as far as is feasible, himself or herself. The old role of passive recipient in care is gone; primary nursing is bringing with it the role of the patient as the active participant and key worker in meeting their own health care needs.

Square pegs in round holes

Despite over a decade of nursing theorists explaining the value of nursing models there remain areas of care where their application has been either slow or non-existent. This section attempts to analyse the reasons for this, and to suggest ways in which movements towards implementation can be facilitated.

Who?	What?	Why?
Where?	When?	Which?

These are all questions which need an answer if the right model is to fit the right patient.

Why?

Why does the situation, defined above, exist in the first place? Surely nurses everywhere recognise the need for a sound philosophical framework for care? Why then are they not turning to the now well-documented nursing theories? Several reasons come to mind. Nursing models, despite the work of Roper, Logan and Tierney (1985), Minshull *et. al.* (1986) and Wright (1986, 1990a) in developing nursing models which are directly relevant to the British nursing arena, are still seen as American (Kershaw and Salvage 1986). In recognising this, Aggleton and Chalmers (1986) and Pearson and Vaughan (1986) made a positive contribution towards ensuring British nurses became aware of their value when applied to care within this country. Occasionally experienced nurses debate their relevance but these debates rarely involve the nurses who have experimented with their use in their own practice setting.

Some of these nurses have explored model-based practice only as part of degree or diploma studies, where students are required to use patient care examples. A few will go on to internalise model-based practice into their own philosophical framework (the aforesaid authors for example), but many more see them as no more than educationally directed exercises. Why have teachers failed to assist practitioners to make the conceptual leap between theory and practice? The reasons for the theory-practice gap are similar regardless of what the theory is and where the practice is meant to be. It is unreasonable, however, to blame the teachers for the situation, just as it is inappropriate to consider the clinical staff responsible for not incorporating new ideas into day-to-day care giving.

One reason, which always comes to the fore in any debate on changes in nursing practice which involve theories and models is that they are 'American'. These arguments are familiar to all nurses, and were applied *ad nauseum* to innovations that involved the nursing process, problem-solving, nursing diagnosis, and primary nursing, to name but a few. They came round, again and again, like a carousel:

'not relevant here'
'won't work'
'nursing here is different'
'health-care is different'
'nurses are different'
'patients don't like it'

The arguments about relevance have been dead for five years, laid to rest with the 1986 publications mentioned earlier which demonstrated application, by nurses, of theories and models through so many varied areas of care. The arguments about health care settings, nursing and nursing being 'different' only apply if you let them. Nursing is different anyway. Contrast for example, an intensive care unit with an elderly sick mentally infirm (ESMI) day hospital; or a health centre with night duty on an acute medical ward. Nurses differ depending on their training, their socialisation, their experiences since registration, and their individual philosophy on life; one doesn't need to cross oceans to know that! Surely the caring principles which underpin competent, professional practice are common to all, and nurses are intelligent enough to make the conceptual jumps which allow them to introduce model based practice. Why they have not been introduced cannot be because nurses don't recognise their value, or because they aren't seen as relevant to practice here. More realistic reasons for non-introduction must be looked for. We'll return to the real reasons for this later.

There are also those who suggest that patients' relatives may not like model based practice. I would argue that this excuse is not only unfounded, but that we are using it as an excuse not to meet our responsibilities towards patients/clients. Patients do not like many of the activities we force upon them when they enter health care settings. Entry into the patient role can be traumatic, taking away individualism, choice and maturity. But nurses, doctors and other health care workers persist in ensuring patients appreciate the need for their actions, the necessity for them to co-operate with care and treatment regimes by convincing them that this is the way to positive health adaptation.

Brearley (1990) recognises that patients need to participate, preferring to be involved and consulted. He also acknowledges that they appreciate care which is structured and logically delivered. If they had a choice, would they not prefer care-giving to be based on a sound theoretical framework than ritualistically? (Walsh and Ford 1989). Wright, whose work in developing and implementing model-based practice clearly demonstrated how valuable it is for patients to feel involved in the care planning, also showed how effective that care partnership is when delivered in an environment with a common nursing philosophy/model. He has, more recently, taken model-based practice further by linking it to primary nursing.

Of course, there are many nurses like Wright who will continue to find it difficult to take someone else's model on board and use it directly in their own practice area. I am one of those myself, preferring to explore several different curriculum models and adapt them to my own philosophical framework. The individual in me, the 'uniqueness' of my college and our clinical units, the special nature of my colleagues all make this adaptation and revision essential. No-one needs to be afraid to adapt and revise any model for their own use. Precedents have been set and are widely published in the United Kingdom. The essential nature of adapting a model for one's own use must lie in ensuring congruence with all other nurses involved in caring for the patients and family. Perhaps the real reason why nurses have not been able to introduce model-based practices as they would wish lies in the time needed to achieve this congruence (Wright, 1986, Pearson and Vaughan, 1986). Introducing any change takes time and time is what nurses in the 1990s have little of. Pressure for change, in so many areas, is being forced upon us. Something which needs such preparation as this does will inevitably become a victim to the pressures of a modern day in the ward or community centre. Only when managers recognise the value of model-based care will nurses receive the assistance necessary to introduce it. The contracts and quality work within the

White Papers of recent years may yet turn out to be supporting the process of change.

Who?

The person who has the key responsibility for the introduction must be the ward sister, the G grade post-holder, supported by the nurse and non-nurse managers, and assisted by the educational staff. Some units will be fortunate enough to have specialist practitioners, but most will be on their own. Attempts should be made to ensure the co-operation of the medical staff. Doctors are now much more receptive to innovative nursing care, especially when it aids recovery, facilitates early discharge, and reduces re-admission. Their anxiety about nurses interfering in treatment regimes is reducing as nurses become skilled in advocacy and in explaining their actions. Many nurses are actively involved in working with doctors and other health-care workers within the multi-disciplinary team. Such co-operation can only aid integration and the development of new ideas.

Medical practice too is changing. Increasingly doctors are recognising the value of permanent adaptation, of encouraging co-operation, of working towards independence and of self-help. These are all recognisable as key concepts of model-based practice. Some medical regimes, such as insulin therapy, chemotherapeutic and radiotherapeutic regimes and active rehabilitation programmes, are much more effective if patients co-operate and are involved in their care and treatment planning (Brearley, 1990). Nurses and doctors, working together with occupational therapists, dieticians and family members can co-ordinate care positively. Model-based practice can help.

Finally, if you are fortunate enough to have specialist nursing support, use it, but don't let it control you or the change process. Remember, you are responsible and accountable for ensuring that your patients receive what you believe is the best possible standard of care. If you believe that this is best achieved by introducing model-based practice it is you who need to introduce it!

Why?

Walsh (1990) sees model-based care as challenging traditional ritualistic practice, bringing new approaches to care and making nursing more accountable to patients and their families. Henderson (1990) defines model based practice as 'a framework, a guide, a structured way to plan, implement and evaluate care'. This is, of course, not to say all these objectives cannot be achieved without model-based practice. Perhaps though, they might be achieved quicker with it!

As seen earlier, if you believe that model-based practice is best for your patients you have a professional obligation to introduce it, as far as is feasible and practicable. At the very least you need to be able to demonstrate that the care you give, and that which is given by those who work with you and for you, is based on sound nursing concepts and a recognised knowledge base. It is insufficient to plan care based on doctors' orders, or Walsh's nursing rituals. Model-based practice recognises the quality of research findings, and encourages their application to practice, invariably based on the core concepts of physiology, psychology and sociology. Many nursing models acknowledge the scientific basis for medical care and treatment, whilst others explore philosophical perspectives.

Many more nurses are using the nursing process/problem-solving approach than are using nursing models. The two do however, 'go together' and interlink very comfortably. They do enable us to be seen as clearly accountable for the quality of the care we give, which is a necessity in these days of contracting and purchaser/provider units.

Where?

Model-based practice needs to be introduced into a receptive, supportive environment, in which the sister is received as and recognised as a competent, professional practitioner. Model-based practice can also be introduced in stages, a few patients at a time, as part of a planned programme with the prior consultation of all concerned. Model-based practice can be introduced in any clinical environment, provided the staff are happy with the approach and the manner of the introduction. It is easier to introduce, as we have seen, with supportive management and teaching staff and in units where doctors do not try to control nursing.

There is no evidence to suggest that model-based practice is easier to introduce in a new unit, than an old one, or into a day centre rather than a long-term setting. British literature includes examples of introduction in almost every area of care, and with patients across a wide age-range, and with many and varied conditions needing a totality of medical and surgical interventions. Model-based practice has been introduced in teaching hospitals, in community units, in recognised centres of excellence (such as Nursing Development Units), and in patients' homes (Kershaw and Salvage, 1986; Salvage and Kershaw, 1990; Aggleton and Chalmers 1986). Provided you have the motivation, it is possible to find someone, somewhere who has used it, and is still using it, in a care setting not dissimilar to your own.

When?

'No time like the present'. Having once decided to do it, plan it and get on with it. If the moment is right and everyone is keen to move forward then go ahead and do it. But don't do it at Christmas, over the summer holiday period, immediately prior to, or following, the appointment of a new manager or at the same time as the College of Nursing is introducing project 2000 with all the changes that will bring. Whilst on the subject of colleges, never introduce anything because the College, or 'the Board' or indeed anyone else, tells you to. That type of change is doomed to failure.

Which?

The choice is yours; the only constraint being the need to consult, discuss and take your team with you. It is easier to introduce a model that has been tried and tested in this country, if only because you have an example of successful intervention to offer guidance.

How?

The wherewithal to introduce model-based practice lies in an understanding of the change process.

Changing nursing practice. Lancaster and Lancaster (1982) acknowledge that 'many people resist change because of a fear of the unknown'. The primary role of the change-agent must be to remove the anxiety and support the change and the individuals involved throughout the length of the programme.

Becoming a change-agent needs commitment. It is a long-term process, and the individual needs to be able to give the time and energy required. Change-agents need to be knowledgeable and skilled practitioners and they need to be seen as 'part of the team'. In this they differ from a consultancy (a term widely used in NHS settings today) who is invited from without to advise the team but who rarely becomes a full member of it. They need to be at least as equally clinically competent as the team members, and to fully understand the background to the change they are seeking to introduce. This is why directed change from above usually fails in that the change-agent herself has not internalised the knowledge base sufficiently to hold firm when the questions get tough.

As a change agent you need a good reason for wanting to make the change; because you believe it is better than the old way may be sufficient to get *you* started but it won't necessarily carry anyone with you. To do this you need to have explored the background, read what others have successfully achieved, studied why others have failed, and have a convincing argument to support your own plans. You need to involve others in the change so that they too are familiar with the rationale. Discuss your ideas with them, let them criticise and debate your ideas and be prepared to view their commitments constructively even if they are critical. Work out who in your team will support you and who will oppose. In other words, find out who your friends are! Find a good second-in-command, so that the process of change continues when you are not there. You could even consider making someone a key worker, who will perhaps spend more time on the change than you. Your role then becomes that of co-ordinator or adviser.

Set up group discussion while the process is being planned, and while it develops. You can mix those 'for' and 'against' in an attempt to isolate the opposition. Use these groups to impart information as well. Do not be afraid of bringing in outsiders. If the model you want to introduce is being used effectively somewhere else, ask the senior sister to come and talk to your team, or arrange a visit to see her unit in action. Sometimes those from outside are seen as valuable expert advisers, simply because they are not local. Remember 'a prophet is never recognised in his own country'.

Use newsletters, advisory committees, and networks to let everyone know what you plan to do. This saves the 'I didn't know about that' situation, which can be so disruptive and damaging. Finally, acknowledge where you have received help. Make your abstracts and your collection of books available for others to read. If you prepare for change thoroughly, it will be that much easier to introduce.

Introducing change. The steps in introducing change can be clearly defined. Avoid the square peg in the round hole situation by carefully identifying the problem and researching the background alternatives. Then assess the motivation among colleagues. This can be more easily achieved by avoiding surprises. Plan your discussions with them, don't hide what you are *really* doing under the guise of doing something else, and don't blame anyone else for it. It is your idea, your programme, and your plan. Stand up and be counted, admit it, and be proud of it!

It is important to involve senior managers, and get their support if possible. This can usually be achieved by presenting your case as

(a) cost effective
(b) efficient
(c) improving the quality of care
(d) enhancing their position
(e) bringing credit to the organisation

If you cannot get their total support, the least you need is their commitment not to criticise. Bear in mind, though, that change is more difficult to introduce without support. It is important, therefore, to gain some active support, for example, another nurse who is working successfully with models. You could also join the Nursing Development Network, sponsored by the King's Fund Centre. (You will be welcome whether or not you work in a Nursing Development Unit NDU). Use the columns of the nursing press to find like-minded people. You'll be surprised how many deviants there are in nursing once you look!

Information should be provided, but make it relevant and applicable so that you cannot be accused of forcing something on to someone or onto your unit that is not appropriate. It will only work if it is seen as congruent, that is if it fits. Also emphasise any advantages to the staff which will result from the change. Improved patient contact could be one example, while job satisfaction could be another.

It is important to ensure that everyone participates, thus removing the obstacle of square pegs if they exist; also let them feel that some of the ideas are their own. In conceding minor points, which easily outweigh the big issues, you will be seen as taking on board another's ideas. It is helpful to avoid increasing workloads and to recognise that everyone will not be as enthusiastic about the idea as you are. Enthusiasm will be low if, for example, some colleagues have had bad experiences in previous change programmes. Remember to acknowledge each individual's values and ideals; just because they are not the same as yours does not mean you should ignore them.

Finally, don't threaten – this is not the time to suggest 'if you don't like it, go'. (That could come later!) At the beginning, provide support, encouragement and advice.

Leadership. Being a change agent is, of course, all about leadership. Leadership can be defined as providing guidance and direction to others, from a basis of sound professional knowledge and skilled professional practice. It involves support, counselling and teaching, all within a non-threatening environment. This can be a stressful experience, and can make you feel isolated from those you are leading through the change process. At times, you will feel like 'the square peg in the round hole' yourself. Always remember that others have been there before you and go back to your friends, or your network and ask for help and support. Changing practice is all about sharing, and it is too important a responsibility to abdicate the moment the going gets tough. As Sister Plume would have said 'The welfare of our patients is at stake'! (1988–1990).

Table 5.1   Pure essential oils Shirley Price Aromatherapy Limited have a large selection of pure essential oils—over 50—for your use. We have chosen 20 of the most useful ones to tell you about in some detail. Other essential oils on the price list have their uses detailed in our Essential booklet (£1.20 incl. p&p). For further information refer to the book *Practical Aromatherapy* by Shirley Price (£4.25 incl. post and packing).

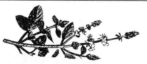

Basil
This oil is produced from the familiar herb used in cooking. It is ideal for revitalising a congested skin. It is uplifting and refreshing and is useful in cases of sinus.

Bergamot
Helpful as a deodorant and can relieve a sore throat, tonsilitis or bad breath. Eases flatulence, indigestion and cystitis.

Chamomile Moroccan
Produced from the wayside plants with the daisy-like flowers, the chamomiles are soothing on all types of skin complaints. Chamomiles are very calming on the nervous system, so will relax a highly emotional person.

Cedarwood
A relaxing oil, good for scalp disorders as well as problems such as cystitis. Sedative.

Clary Sage
From Russia comes this heady oil. Helpful for depression and menstrual problems.

Cypress
Good for menstrual problems, reduces broken and varicose veins and is useful on an oily skin.

Eucalyptus
From the Blue Gum Tree, this oil is excellent for clearing the head and is universally used for colds and bronchial problems. An exhilarating oil, it is also helpful for aches and pains. Good insect repellent.

Fennel
Traditionally used for digestive disorders and together with Dill is used in gripe water for babies.

Frankincense
This ancient oil is wonderfully rejuvenating in skin lotions and creams. Also good for catarrh and other mucous conditions.

Geranium
The greenish oil from the Bourbon Isles has an exquisite sweet aroma. Used in the bath it is relaxing to the body and refreshing to the mind. Geranium also helps to clear dry eczema or dermatitis and is ideal for an oily skin.

Juniper
Both stimulating and relaxing, it helps to clear skin and scalp problems. It is also helpful to the kidneys, and an invaluable aid against fluid retention.

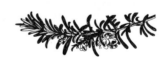

Lavender
The most versatile, all round oil, suitable for all skin types and very good for various skin complaints. It also has calming properties which act on the nervous system as well as relieving headaches, migraines, nose and throat infections and many other ailments. Calms the mind and blends well with other fragrances.

Lemon
Rich with vitamin C and full of zest to enliven. Helpful for sinus conditions and oily or mature skin.

Table 5.1   Pure essential oils – *Continued*

Mandarin
This pleasant oil is uplifting to the spirits. Mild in action it is used in skin care and as a laxative.

Marjoram
Ideal for muscular spasms and sprains, calming, it relieves insomnia, stress and painful periods. Warming and fortifying.

Peppermint
Acts as a natural antiseptic that is calming to an irritated skin. Used in mixtures for headaches, colds and sinusitis. Also very good for stomach disorders.

Rosemary
From the sunny Mediterranean countries this herb has been used for thousands of years. It is invigorating, refreshing, sharpens the memory and enlivens the mind. A cleansing and stimulating oil, good for scalp disorders. Helps relieve cellulite and fluid retention.

Sage
From the well known herb, this useful oil helps clear a congested skin and eases rheumatic conditions. Used to help reduce cellulite and fluid retention.

Sandalwood
This exotic oil from India relieves stress and is good for colic, sore throats and coughs. It is invaluable as an aid to dry skin and eczema conditions.

Ylang-Ylang
A complete oriental perfume in itself, this oil normalises an oily skin. It can induce sleep and is uplifting in cases of depression.

Shirley Price Aromatherapy Ltd., Wesley House, Stockwell Head, Hinckley, Leics. LE10 1RD.

References

Aggleton, P. and Chalmers, H. (1986). *Nursing Models and the Nursing Process*. Macmillan, Basingstoke.

Berman, F. and McLaughlin M. W. (1976). Implementation of educational innovation. *Educational Forum*, **40(3)**, 345–70.

Brearley, S. (1990). *Patient Participation: the Literature*. Scutari, Harrow.

Campbell, A. (1984). *Moderated Love: A Philosophy Of Professional Care*. SPCK, London.

Department of Health (1990). Mrs Bottomley Announces New Charter For Action On Junior Doctors' Hours. DOH, London (Press release H90/616, 17 December).

Elliott-Cannon, C. (1990). Mental handicap and nursing models. In *Models For Nursing 2*, J. Salvage and B. Kershaw (Eds), pp. 77–88. Scutari, London.

Ersser, S. and Tutton, E. (Eds), (1991). *Primary Nursing in Perspective*. Scutari, London.

Goffman, E. (1961). *Asylums*. Penguin, Harmondsworth.

Henderson, C. (1990). Models and midwifery. In *Models For Nursing 2*, J. Salvage and B. Kershaw (Eds), pp. 57–67. Scutari, London.

Henderson, V. (1966). *The Nature of Nursing*. New York, Macmillan.

Johnson, D. E. (1980). The behavioral system model for nursing. In *Conceptual Models For Nursing Practice*. 2nd Edn., J. P. Riehl and C. Roy (Eds), pp. 207–16. Appleton-Century-Crofts, Norwalk.

Kershaw, B. and Salvage, J. (Eds), (1986). *Models For Nursing*. Wiley, Chichester.

Lancaster, J. and Lancaster, W. (1982). *The Nurse As a Change Agent*. Mosby, St Louis.

Manthey, M. (1980). *The Practice Of Primary Nursing*. Blackwell, Boston.

Maslow, A. H. (1970). *Motivation and Personality*. 2nd edn. Harper & Row, New York.

Minshull, J., Ross, K. and Turner, J. (1986). The human needs model of nursing. *Journal of Advanced Nursing*, **11(6)**, 643–9.

Neuman, B. (1982). *The Neuman Systems Model: Application To Nursing Education and Practice*. Appleton-Century-Crofts, Norwalk.

Nightingale, F. (1859). *Notes On Nursing*. Harrison, London.

Orem, D. (1985). *Nursing: Concepts Of Practice*. 3rd edn. McGraw-Hill, New York.

Parse, R. R. (1981). *Man – Living – Health: A Theory Of Nursing*. Wiley, New York.

Pearson, A. and Vaughan, B. (1986). *Nursing Models For Practice*. Heinemann, London.

Pearson, A. (Ed), (1988). *Primary Nursing*. Croom Helm, London.

Riehl-Sisca, J. (1989). The Riehl interaction model: an update. In *Conceptual Models For Nursing Practice*, 3rd edn., J. P. Riehl-Sisca (Ed), pp. 383–402. Appleton and Lange, Norwalk.

Rogers, M. E. (1979). *An Introduction To the Theoretical Basis Of Nursing*. Churchill Livingstone, Edinburgh.

Roper, N., Logan, W. W. and Tierney, A. J. (1985). *The Elements Of Nursing*, 2nd edn. Churchill Livingstone, Edinburgh.

Roy, C. (1984). *Introduction To Nursing: An Adaptation Model*, 2nd edn. Prentice-Hall, Englewood Cliffs.

Salvage, J. and Kershaw, B. (Eds), (1990). *Models For Nursing 2*. Scutari, London.

Sister Plume, (1988–1990). Monthly column in the Nursing Times.

Thibodeau, J. A. (1983). *Nursing Models: Analysis and Evaluation*. Wadsworth, Monterey.

Waldegrave, W. (1991). Presentation on 20th May at the Royal College of Nursing Annual Congress. Unpublished.

Walsh, M. and Ford, P. (1989). *Nursing Rituals, Research and Rational Actions*. Heinemann, Oxford.

Walsh, M. (1990). From model to care plan. In *Models For Nursing 2*. J. Salvage and B. Kershaw (Eds), pp. 39–45. Scutari, London.

Watson, J. (1979). *The Philosophy and Science Of Caring*. Little, Brown, Boston.

World Health Organization, (1946). *Constitution of the World Health Organization*. WHO, Geneva.

Wright, S. G. (1986). *Building and Using A Model Of Nursing*. Edward Arnold, London.

Wright, S. G. (1990a). *Building and Using A Model Of Nursing*. 2nd edn. Edward Arnold, London.

Wright, S. G. (1990b). *My Patient – My Nurse*. Scutari, London.

Suggested further reading

Fawcett, J. (1990). *An Analysis and Evaluation Of Conceptual Models In Nursing*. 2nd edn. Philadelphia, FA Davis.

George, J. (Ed). (1980). *Nursing Theories: The Base For Professional Nursing*. 2nd edn. Practice. Prentice-Hall, New Jersey.

Kenney, J. (1990). Theory-based nursing practice. In *Nursing Process: Application Of Conceptual Models*, P. Christensen and J. Kenney, (Eds). C. V. Mosby, St Louis.

Nyatanga, L. (1990). Nursing paradigm: the state of the art. *Senior Nurse* **10(4)**, pp. 18–19.

Selanders, L. and Dietz-Omour, M. (1991). Making nursing models relevant for the practising nurse. *Nursing Practice/NS*, **4(2)**, 23–25.

6 Information systems in modern nursing

It is probably true to say that nurses throughout the last 100 years, at least, have considered their nursing practice to be 'modern' and up-to-date. Changes in nurse training have taken place. These changes, and those in nursing practice, have resulted from new nursing knowledge and advances in medical practice. The latest ideas are often considered an improvement on past practice.

Since the National Health Service (NHS) came into being in 1948 nurse training has been nationally monitored and controlled. Despite this, practice and standards of nursing care are not equal on a national basis. As the NHS has grown, so the management of it has become more complex. No longer are individual hospitals run by matrons and medical directors. When the NHS was re-organised in 1979 hospitals were grouped together as part of District Health Authorities (DHA). Since then, hospitals have been run by managers in the DHA. Everyone working in the NHS today is part of a very large organisation employing about one million people, nearly half of whom are nurses. Today's management structures are often large and complex. The effective management of health services is dependent upon managers making important and informed decisions about the use of resources; human, material, financial and informational.

Managers need to monitor and control the use of these resources within the organisation, and in order to do this they need to have:

(*i*)   a clear idea of what ought to be occurring
(*ii*) a good idea of what is actually happening
(*iii*) some means of correcting any discrepancy.

In order to manage effectively managers need **reliable, relevant** and **recent** information upon which to base their decisions. These could be considered the 3Rs of information:

(a)   **reliable information** which is based on data collected carefully using a reliable data collection method. **Rubbish in = rubbish out (!!)**.
(b)   **relevant information** which informs them about the situation and is not cluttered with other irrelevant facts.

138

(c)   **recent information** which has been generated from data collected in the not too distant past and is based on current or recent events or changes.

Data (plural of datum) are the raw materials, the symbols and patterns, from which information can be derived. A computer works only with data.

Information is analyzed or processed data. Data becomes information only when it has been structured in such a way that it is meaningful to the user. For example, the digits 022778 could be an STD code, a date or an invoice number. The digits do not represent a date unless it is also known that the user required the information in the order of month, day and year. It is essential for items of data to be **related** to each other to represent the information that users need. The following questions need to be borne in mind:

- Where does information come from?
- Where does information go?
- Who uses the information?
- What is an information system?
- Who needs, or has access to, the information?

Information needs to be generated and disseminated throughout the organisation, quickly, efficiently, reliably and accurately. The system used for this purpose today will most probably be computerised. A **computer-based information system** is an information system where the computer is an integral part of the system and provides for the flow and storage of information. Many computer-based information systems are used by managers of health care. These systems include **nursing information systems**. The information generated from such a system is an integral part of a **health care information system** and will be considered in that context.

Although computer technology has been used in hospital environments for over 20 years, it is only recently that the nursing profession has begun to realise its potential value for nursing practice. Nursing has now begun to view computer technology as a necessary resource. (Cox *et. al.*, 1987)

A nursing information system can be used for patient care management and for the management of resources related to nursing care delivery. Nursing information systems can also provide data bases that can be used for research, policy and decision-making processes. It is essential, therefore, that nurses acquire the knowledge and skills to enable them effectively to use the technology. They will need to be computer literate and to have a knowledge of economic and business principles to enable them to participate in budget planning, costing, financial and information management. (Perrin, 1990)

Information technology

Although computers are a relatively recent invention the development of this technology, especially the silicon chip (microchip), has resulted in enormous advances in the use and range of information technology (IT). IT is the generic term used to describe the processing of information using microprocessor-based electronic equipment. At the heart of the computer is the central processing unit (CPU) which logically obeys program instructions. The CPU operates inputs and/or stored data to produce outputs or other stored data (see list of abbreviations, page 169).

Computer hardware

This refers to the computer itself which may be large (mainframe), mini (smaller) or micro (smallest). Hardware includes the peripheral equipment needed to run computer programs.

Input devices – keyboard (computer or musical), mouse, tracker ball, bar code reader, light pen, scanner, electronic pen, touch screen, voice activation machine and modem.

Output devices – printer, visual display unit (VDU), speech synthesis and modem.

Data storage systems – floppy disc, hard disc (Winchester), audio tape, tape streamer, laser disc or CD-ROM (Compact Disc – Read Only Memory) and EPROM (Erasable Programmable Read Only Memory). *See* Fig. 6.1.

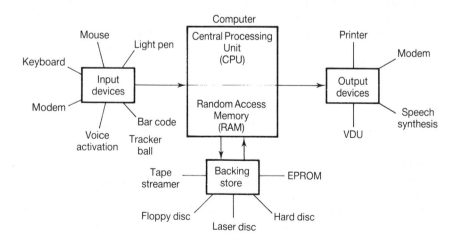

Fig. 6.1   A computer system (A. Trueman, 1991)

Computer memory

One type of computer memory is RAM (random access memory). This is the normal working area of the computer. RAM is transient; it can be written to, can store data and previously stored data can be read from it. However, it requires a steady power source to retain the memory. It can easily be over-written or destroyed and is lost completely when power is removed.

Home micro computers have from 32k to 32mb of RAM. A 'k' is a kilobyte or about 1000 characters. An Acorn BBC Model B computer, for example, has 32k of RAM, the Master 128 has 128k, the Archimedes up to 4mb of RAM and IBM 'compatibles' have up to 32 megabytes (mb) or 32,000k of RAM. In a mainframe computer the RAM is measured in gigobytes (gb). Most hospital information systems would need a mainframe computer to cope with their data requirements.

The other type of computer memory is ROM (read only memory). This consists of silicon 'chips'. They contain sets of instructions or programs that actually 'tell' the computer what to do in response to certain key words or phrases (syntax). The memory capacity of ROMs is 8k to 500k. More modern versions of ROMs, not based on silicon are being introduced into IT, CD-ROMs being the most common.

Computer software

Software is the name given to instructions or programs that 'tell' the computer what to do. Each type of computer uses its own language (syntax). This language, for example MS-DOS (Microsoft – Disc Operating System), can either be resident on a chip (ROM) inside the computer, or it may be supplied on disc to be loaded into the computer each time it is used.

Data storage systems

Programs and work (files) can be temporarily stored in RAM. Once the power is switched off, or another program loaded, all the data (and hard work!) can be lost. There has to be a way of storing and retrieving data or programs that is readily accessible and secure. These include:

1. **Floppy discs** which are made of magnetic material. They are usually 3.5″ or 5.25″ in diameter and can store 300k to 1.4mb on each one. They are cheap but are slow in access time and they suffer badly under high usage and poor storage conditions.
2. **Hard discs**, often known as Winchesters, which have massive

storage capacities, 10mb to 1000mb, are much faster to access. These are much more expensive and are costly to backup.

3. **CD-ROMs** are based on the 5.25″ laser compact disc (CD). A typical laser disc can hold 540mb. Two would hold the whole of Encyclopaedia Britannica and CD-ROMs can provide databases, references and other information for libraries, replacing the need for vast shelves of reference books. The advantage of ROM is that it is more or less permanent and does not require power to maintain its state. Databases can be kept up to date cheaply and efficiently by sending the library the latest version of the CD-ROM.

4. **Tape streamers** which are used to store vast amounts of data, often to back up the data on a mainframe computer.

There are several applications of Information Technology (IT) in office and management areas such as word processing, spreadsheets, databases and graphics.

Word processing is used by many organisations to produce letters and documents. The advantage of a word processor over normal typing is that documents can be typed in as normal, spelling checked, the format designed for the page on the screen, stored on disc and later retrieved and amended without the whole document having to be re-typed.

Spreadsheets enable data to be set up and calculations made of a 'what if?' nature on the computer. The information is presented in a tabular or grid format and is especially useful in resource management.

Databases are a method of storing large amounts of information defined by the user. They are used to retrieve information quickly on a selective basis. A **patient master index (PMI)** as part of **patient administration systems (PAS)** is a good example of a database in a hospital information system.

Image processing/Graphics enable data to be displayed in a graphical form (line, bar or pie chart) and incorporated in a word processed document, if required. **Facsimile machines (FAX)** are an example of images (data) being transferred via a telephone with the receiver obtaining a printout of the information sent.

Desktop publishing (DTP) can be thought of as a combination of word processing and graphics. Applications of this range from simple production of posters or leaflets to the design and layout of a complete manual.

Statistical analysis can be undertaken by the computer which is capable of carrying out many complex calculations. An example of this is the Health Service Indicators (HSIs) produced annually by the Department of Health (DoH) from data collected by health authorities.

Expert systems can be used as an electronic reference book, for example, to aid doctors in diagnosis and treatment selection.

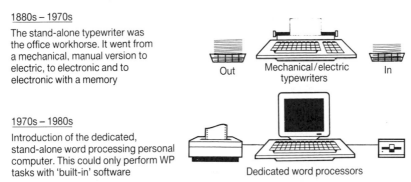

1880s – 1970s

The stand-alone typewriter was the office workhorse. It went from a mechanical, manual version to electric, to electronic and to electronic with a memory

Out   Mechanical/electric typewriters   In

1970s – 1980s

Introduction of the dedicated, stand-alone word processing personal computer. This could only perform WP tasks with 'built-in' software

Dedicated word processors

Fig. 6.2 Evolution of IT 1870s–1980s (Evans, 1990)

Information systems

One computer on its own, although capable of handling vast amounts of data, does not constitute an information system. Once data have been collected, processed and stored, information can be generated. This information may be very useful to the user but, if it is to be communicated and made available to others within and without the organisation, there needs to be a system of connections. Such systems include:

1. **Computer networking** which consists of a number of computers inter-connected and inter-communicating in some way. If all the computer hardware in the network is of a similar type and manufacture, then networking may be quite simple. Networking is sometimes applied to computer terminals linked to a mainframe computer. An example of this is a PAS.
2. **A File server** which is a 'memory box' which holds the operating software, applications packages and user files.
3. **Local Area Network (LAN)** which is a computer network covering a small area, such as a group of offices on the same site. Users can transmit and receive messages from other users, access files on the file server and can communicate with remote fax, printing, Prestel, telephone or telex services.
4. **Wide Area Network (WAN)**, as its name implies, applies to a larger computer network system.
5. **Modems** which are devices that can link computers via a telephone line, so that data can be transmitted at high speeds over long distances, nationally and internationally, if required.
6. **Electronic messaging systems** which include terms like **computer based messaging systems (CBMS)** or **computer mediated communication (CMC)**.

7. **Electronic mail** which enables the user to send a message electronically to the mailbox of another user, perhaps via a modem or the LAN/WAN system. Mailboxes are like electronic desks to which and from which messages can be sent, stored and read. Each mailbox user's electronic address is unique.

8. **Bulletin board systems (BBS)** which are the simplest form of CMC. Of the large public on-line services, the principal system is Prestel with some 300 000 pages of information and hundreds of information providers. Prestel is widely used in the field of travel, banking and the stock exchange. A second major on-line service is Telecom Gold. This system carries electronic mail, a BBS and extensive file facilities. In 1987 the Open Software Library (OSL) set up a specialist BBS for health care workers. This can be accessed via a modem, all for the cost of a phone call. Access can be restricted to some of the databases held on BBS by the use of codes or user identification (ID) numbers.

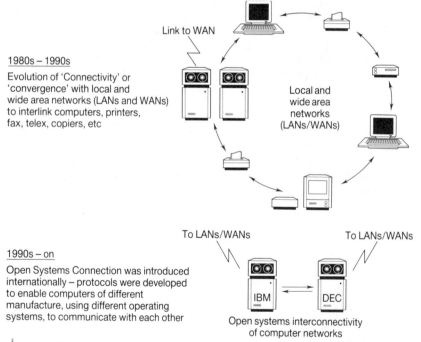

Link to WAN

1980s – 1990s

Evolution of 'Connectivity' or 'convergence' with local and wide area networks (LANs and WANs) to interlink computers, printers, fax, telex, copiers, etc

Local and wide area networks (LANs/WANs)

To LANs/WANs   To LANs/WANs

1990s – on

Open Systems Connection was introduced internationally – protocols were developed to enable computers of different manufacture, using different operating systems, to communicate with each other

IBM   DEC

Open systems interconnectivity of computer networks

Fig. 6.3   Evolution of IT 1980s to the present day (Evans, 1990)

A word of warning!

Just because information has been obtained from a computer there is no guarantee that it is correct! Remember the rubbish in = rubbish out phenomenon? **Nurses should not** be afraid to question information generated by a computerised information system. The information will only be as reliable as the data from which it has been generated, and the person/people who put in the data. Computer networks provide a facility to spread *wrong* information over a wide area, with the associated potential for an ensuing disaster.

Health care information systems

The NHS/DHSS Steering Group on Health Service Information, under the chairmanship of Edith Körner, produced the Körner Reports between 1982 and 1984. Each of these covered a major area of NHS activity on which national, regional and local management needed to collect information. These included hospital facilities, diagnostic services, paramedical services, community services, manpower, finance and patient transport. Collection of Körner data on patient activity and hospital facilities began in April 1987, with data from community and paramedical services following a year later.

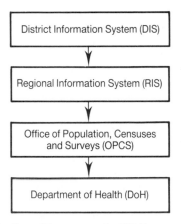

Fig. 6.4 Körner data flow (Trueman, A. 1991)

Districts are required to collect **minimum data sets (MDS)** on each area of activity. Most MDS occur as a natural by-product of operational computer systems. Districts use a **Patient Administration System (PAS)** to collect the data they require for the Körner central requirements, storing it on a **District Information System (DIS)**. Information on the DIS is then sent to region, which gathers information from all its districts onto a **Regional Information System (RIS)**. Once a quarter the relevant information is sent by tape to the **Office of Population, Censuses and Surveys (OPCS)** which prepares monthly and annual reports for the **Department of Health (DoH)**. The DoH uses the data for many purposes. The main one is for Health Service Indicators. These provide information on the work done by health authorities, the staff they employ and the resources they use. HSIs were developed to help authorities to monitor and plan the delivery of services, and to help them to assess how they compare with others in a national setting.

Resource management in health services

Health care delivery and the planning of services is based on the 'needs' of various groups within the population. The concept of 'need' is difficult to define. Kalino (1979) cited by Rathwell (1987; p. 101) defines need as 'the difference between observed and ideal levels of health'. People generally desire the best health care available but may be unwilling to pay more for it, or to take responsibility for their own state of health. The known relationship between smoking and lung cancer does not, appear to deter many people from smoking.

The effective planning and control of resources should result in better value from available resources and the provision of a better service for patients. Managers, including clinicians and nurses, need information to enable them to take decisions and to make informed judgements to achieve maximum effective use and control of resources. Since 1984 there have been a number of changes introduced by Government involving increased decentralisation of decision making. This has been matched by increasing pressure for up-to-date information, particularly at operational level.

The Griffiths Report (NHS Management Inquiry Team, 1983) recommended management arrangements which focus upon clearly accountable **general managers**. Decentralisation only works properly when there is sufficient information to monitor performance of the tasks which have been devolved. Griffiths recommended the design and implementation of management budgeting, and demonstration sites were then set up. In the light of experience gained from these demonstration sites the **Resource Management Initiative (RMI)** was announced at the end of 1986, with the objective of promoting effectiveness and efficiency in the **National Health Service (NHS)**. RMI was designed to tackle the problem of controlling those resources used by professionals in providing care for patients. (National Health Service Management Executive, 1990a) Doctors and nurses would be encouraged to participate actively in the management process, and managers would be supported by information systems which are capable of costing the services provided to each patient.

Resource management (RM) is a way of organising the resources of a unit by increasing the involvement of all the clinical staff in its management. This will provide them with more accurate and useful information about their clinical practice and its cost, enabling them to compare with colleagues in other units in the same hospital, district, or region. There is a need to link and relate patient activity data to the costs of running the service. Doctors, nurses and paramedics need to be involved in designing periodic reports and in making use of the resultant information.

Budgets are related to workload for individual or groups of service providers and the responsibility for each budget given to an individual manager. Some hospitals are adopting a clinical directorate model where consultant staff are assigned to a 'directorate' based on broad specialty groupings. One person, usually a consultant, is appointed as director for a term of office. The director is assigned a budget and has managerial accountability for resources used by the directorate. This may also include all the staff assigned to it. Devolved decision making and budgeting, arising from resource management information systems has many implications, for both the senior nurse manager and, ultimately, the ward sister. In some directorates the ward sister is the nursing budget manager, while in others it may be a senior nurse or a non-nurse.

Resource management in the NHS can only be achieved by the active involvement of clinicians and nurses in the management process. Managers need to be supported by information systems which are capable of costing the services provided by each patient. Doctors generally commit resources through their clinical judgement, whereas nurses actually deliver the major part of care to patients. In order for clinical staff to begin to be involved in managing the resources which they commit to the provision of patient care, various information inputs need to be made. The information required if the clinician is to manage effectively includes:

(a) plans for future level of service and likely resource requirements.
(b) budget and resources allocated to provide a given level of service.
(c) how the resources have been managed to achieve the required level of service.
(d) regular monitoring of the service provision and resource use.
(e) a review of the service use and value.

The White Paper proposals (Department of Health, 1989) can be seen as an attempt to speed up the process of change set in motion by these earlier reforms. The current proposals incorporate the earlier initiatives such as general management, strategic information systems and resource management. Since April 1st, 1991 implementation of the White Paper has resulted in a limited trading environment in which patients can receive service by travelling to other places. This is designed to stimulate competition and to accelerate the pace of change. By separating the **purchaser's** role (of assessing the needs of the population, setting up contracts and paying for services as they are used) from the role of **providing** services the process of devolution is being further encouraged. Both purchasers and providers will become increasingly dependent on reliable, relevant and recent information. Purchasers will need to:

(a)   **plan** the procurement of health services in order to arrive at a strategic plan capable of addressing the needs of the resident population. This overall plan will be expressed within a series of annual operational plans.

(b)   **implement** the short term plans by acquiring funding and by negotiating a range of contracts capable of delivering the required range of services. It will be important to quantify the gap between what can be paid for, and what is needed.

(c)   **manage** the contracts once agreed, including the receipt and payment of invoices from various suppliers, and capturing information on the services provided and their outcomes.

(d)   **monitor and report** on the performance of suppliers and of itself as purchaser in terms of contracts, outcomes, changes in health status of the population and the measurement of unmet needs.

(e)   **collect and maintain** the base data required to perform the above tasks.

The White Paper places a clear responsibility upon Health Authorities to measure the needs of their population. The principal tool required for this is a geo-demographic database. Having measured the needs of the population with geo-demographic tools, the gap between provision and need must be identified by comparing needs with information on how the service is being and has been used.

Providers of services will need very detailed clinically based management information, clearly referenced to individual patients, and containing both accurate and comprehensive diagnostic and treatment data. This detailed information will be used to support **medical audit** and to establish control costs. White Paper changes will also require support contracts with Community Service agencies to be drawn up. General practitioners (GPs) with practices serving seven thousand patients or more will have the option of managing their own budgets. These GPs are known as fund holders (GPFH).

Providers, whether Directly Managed Units (DMUs) or NHS Trusts must, from April 1st, 1991, be able to set prices; assess demand from their local catchment population; have contractual arrangements with buyers; be able to negotiate contracts; account for services rendered and invoice for them; have an asset register; provide annual accounts and provide data for nationally defined purposes. To be able to do this appropriate information systems are necessary. All providers, including NHS Trusts, will have an obligation to supply data for national registers such as the Cancer Registry. National registers form a very important data source for public health and outcome measures.

The implementation of resource management is one of the essential conditions for hospitals before they are allowed to become self-governing under the White Paper proposals. These hospitals will need the information systems to cost treatments and to monitor their budgets. The roles of purchaser and provider call for information exchange on a large scale. This will result in the use of information technology for most activities within a health district and the replacement of paper records by electronic ones.

Information systems and IT are rapidly becoming essential tools in almost every area of the NHS. At one time a computer system could be installed in one area, without any regard for its wider environment. Now interaction and communication between information systems are not just desirable, they are essential if new management systems, processes and functions are to reach the levels of sophistication and efficiency which the NHS must achieve in a modern world. (National Health Service Information Management Group/Department of Health, 1990). Computer systems in the different parts of the NHS, and from different suppliers, will increasingly need to communicate with, and be compatible with, each other. Information from GP to the DoH and back, as shown in Fig. 6.5 demonstrates a flow of health service information.

A framework used for the evaluation of health services (Donabedian, 1966 cited by Willis and Linwood, 1984) can also be used as a framework (Table 6.1) for identifying areas where management information is needed and information systems can be used. For example:

1. **Structure/input information** on the material, financial and human resources needed and available (the health care setting)
2. **Process information** on the carrying out of care, using the resources, that is the provision of care which constitutes the service
3. **Outcome information** on the efficiency and effectiveness of the care given, **the outputs and the outcomes**.

Structure information

This is by far the largest amount of information which will be available and needed by health service managers. Geo-demographic information is needed from which providers and purchasers of health services can forecast the likely health care needs of a given population. Information is needed about available resources/assets, both material and human. Information is also needed on numbers and types of

Fig. 6.5 Flow of health service information

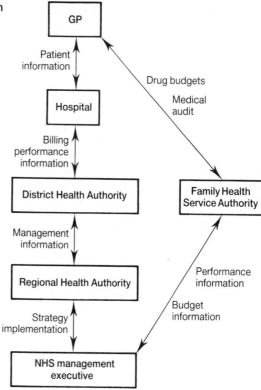

Table 6.1 Information Framework

Structure information	Process information	Outcome/output information
Equipment	Methods of care delivery	Measuring what happens to
Buildings	Care plans:	the patient in terms of:
CSSD	Assessment procedure	health status, level of self-
DISS	Appropriateness of	care, comfort, pain
Staff numbers	intervention	Morbidity
Staff grade	Evaluating level of	Mortality
Skill mix	competence	PIs
Policies	Monitoring systems and	Minimum Data
Data protection	equipment	Sets (MDS)
PAS	WNMIS	
DIS	Medical and nursing	
HIS	workload	
PMI	Drugs	
	Laboratory and other tests	
	Expert systems	

patients (potential and actual), who will be using the services. These all need to be accounted for in financial terms.

A computer-based system using a modular approach has been suggested by the White Paper Working Party on Project 34 to provide a District Information Support System (DISS). This system would include a planning database, invoice processing facilities, contract management and management information. The structure information can be further divided into information on potential and actual patients, manpower requirements and finance.

Patient information

Information on potential and actual patients within a population can be obtained through the DISS planning database. This is a demographic database which is capable of analysing the structure of local populations. This would indicate mortality, morbidity and socio-economic data and will involve collaboration with GPs, local authorities and voluntary agencies. Postcoding will be the key element and the database will depend on the population register derived from the Family Health Service Authority (FHSA). (Up to September 1990 this was known as the Family Practitioner Committee (FPC)).

One way of relating patients to a particular cost centre is to classify the patient by **diagnosis related group (DRG)**. DRGs provide a way of classifying acute, non-psychiatric in-patients according to diagnoses, operations, age, sex, and discharge status. There are 467 different DRGs to cover the range of patients seen in acute hospitals.

Once a patient has been referred to hospital by his GP his name and details will be entered on the **patient master index (PMI)** (sometimes called a **master patient index (MPI)**, which is part of the **patient administration system (PAS)**). In the future patients may have a health card, also known as a Smart Card (Figure 6.6), generated from the

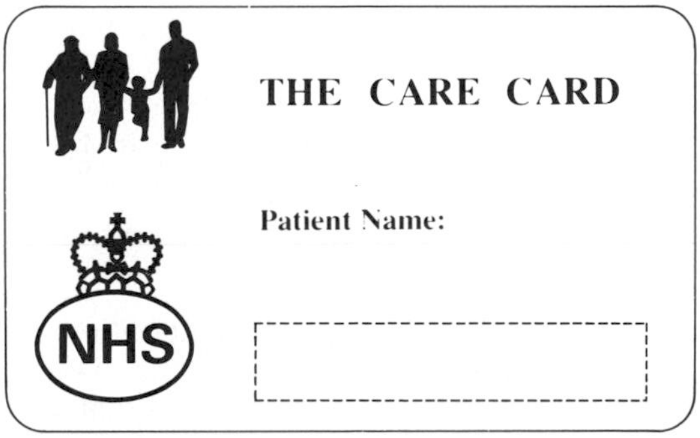

THE CARE CARD

Patient Name:

NHS

Fig. 6.6 Care card

computer system in the GP practice, which contains all his health information. Similar to a credit card, data can be read from an electronic strip by a card reader. Access would be granted to authorised persons such as doctors, dentists, pharmacists and other health care professionals (Fig. 6.7).

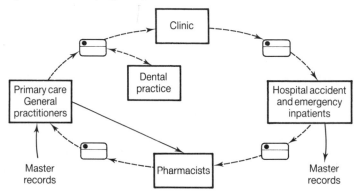

Fig. 6.7   Care card – efficiency in health care (National Health Service, 1989)

A **hospital information system (HIS)**, which would include the PMI and PAS, can collect details of every intervention made during an episode of patient care. For example, every ward and clinic based task can be covered by the system. Doctors can prescribe drugs, order any medical service, test or investigation and view results.

During hospitalisation a **ward nursing management information system (WNMIS)** can record all nursing documentation, care planning and acuity measurements so that the patient record contains a complete and detailed record of interventions made. Handwritten notes are needed only for doctors' clinical commentary. Profiles of the normal workload of specialties, or of individual clinicians, can be constructed, costed and used as a basis for case-mix costing and budgeting systems. The reliability of information created from a case-mix, or other database, depends on data integrity and the timeliness of data input. Some districts have a database co-ordinator whose job it is to check data quality and to resolve any inconsistent data.

Manpower information

The most valuable resources within an organisation are its human resources, and their value increases over time. Human resources management includes planning to meet future manpower needs. Nurse manpower planning means planning for the right numbers of nurses, with the right skills, to be in the right place at the right time.

Many factors affect the number of nursing staff required at any one time, including the numbers of patients and their levels of dependency on nursing staff, the medical and nursing policies being followed and the availability of support staff.

Nurses form the largest group in the NHS, 40–50 per cent of the total NHS workforce. Nurses account for up to 60 per cent of the workforce in some hospitals. Decisions on the numbers and types of nurses to employ may be based on output and outcome information produced at ward level. This will be discussed further in the section on process information.

Computerised staff personnel records, including those of nurses, are usually held centrally and have restricted access. If information systems are to be fully integrated some personnel data will need to link with the nursing information system at ward level. Managers need reliable information on which to make decisions on nursing establishments and recruitment needs. A basic objective of nurse manpower planning is to match the demand with the supply of nursing staff.

Finance information

The **Financial Information Project (FIP)**, based in the West Midlands RHA, has sought to bring together information on activity, manpower, and finance, in a single or integrated information system. Its most publicised work has been in information systems for ward nursing, for operating theatres and for community services. An example of such an operating theatre system is ORSOS (Operating Room Scheduling Office System) details of which are shown in Appendix 1.

Providers of health services will need computerised invoice processing facilities – including a system to validate and authorise payments for services provided.

Process information

Clinical ward managers need information to enable them to manage nursing and other resources effectively. Good, relevant information is essential to the planning and monitoring of effectively delivered, high quality patient care. Nursing information systems are a key element in the resource management programme. (NHSME, August 1990) The availability of a **ward nursing management information system (WNMIS)** can provide nurses with a computerised ward-based system. Data from the **patient administration system (PAS)** and **patient master index (PMI)** can be networked with the WNMIS. Patient details such as name, age, address, etc. would normally be generated externally to the ward. Detailed information can then be collected about the services used per patient. From this information the cost per case can be calculated and charged back to the cost centre. The provision of quality individualised nursing care in a safe environment includes the following:

(i)   setting standards
(ii)   planning individual patient care
(iii) monitoring and evaluating patient care and the environment
(iv)   co-ordinating services to the patient

The documentation of a systematic approach to patient care which involves patient assessment, objective/goal setting, nursing interventions and evaluation of care will provide a nursing record. The patient and the nurse(s) giving care, provide information for the nursing record. Much of the information about patients will, therefore, be generated at ward level. Once targets for the clinical areas have been identified and agreed, planning and managing resources involves the following:

(a)   identification of staff workload and skill mix requirements.
(b)   deployment of suitably skilled staff.
(c)   effective deployment of allocated resources.
(d)   efficient use of all resources.
(e)   collaboration with other departments and professions.
(f)   monitoring and ordering services/supplies.
(g)   reports on ward, patient and staff activity, i.e. outputs and outcomes.

Much of the output/outcome information will form the basis of structure information for the future. If nursing resources are to be deployed effectively clinical ward managers need to know how much nursing care is needed by each patient, or group of patients. Much effort has been invested in estimating and planning the demand for nursing staff. There are two approaches which are commonly used:

(a) Patient/nurse dependency, which relies on the classification of patients and allocating them to a dependency category. Patients are classified using pre-determined averaged workload measurements, which take into account professionally and locally agreed timings for nursing interventions. Workload measurements should translate into nursing hours and skill mix required for groups of patients. Nursing dependency information 'will assist not only in clinical budgeting, but also in helping plan, monitor and control staffing of hospitals in terms of numbers, skills and grades of nurses needed overall, and on individual wards to balance the goals of meeting patient needs relative to economy in nursing costs' (Perrin, 1990; p. 175).

(b) Activity analyses, which are based on records of the actual nursing interventions required by each patient at the time of the patient's assessment and care planning. Productive and non-productive time needs to be taken into account when calculating nursing workload. Information on the hours and skills of nurses actually deployed is also needed to identify any discrepancies between actual and planned deployment. Nursing numbers and skill mix may be determined on the basis of retrospective or prosepective workload information. Once the numbers of nurses and their skill mix have been determined clinical ward managers need manpower and personnel information to enable them to plan for the efficient and effective deployment of available staff. Information on costs will help to ensure that planning is within budget limits.

Staff personnel records are usually held outside the ward, some-times on other systems, which may or may not be networked to the WNMIS. If allocated ward staff, trained and untrained, are to be effectively deployed at ward level, an accurate and flexible computerised ward rostering system is a great advantage. Patient workload information can be incorporated into some systems to help managers to meet nurse/patient workload requirements.

Nurses are not the only professionals involved with patient care. Other health care professionals, such as doctors, physiotherapists, occupational therapists, and others may also contribute to the ward-

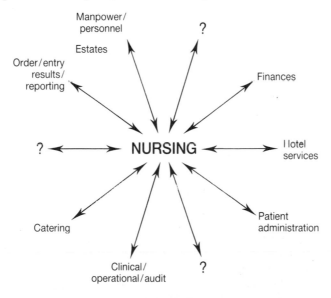

? = other information interchanges

Fig. 6.8   Nursing – information exchanges (National Health Service Management Executive, 1990b)

based records on patient care. Nursing, via the WNMIS, will eventually have links with other parts of the district information system leading to an exchange of information within the system. The identified benefits of using information from a computerised information system include better patient care, best use of nursing and other resources which, in turn, leads to improved job satisfaction for nurses. Figure 6.9 summarises these benefits. (National Health Service Management Executive, 1990b)

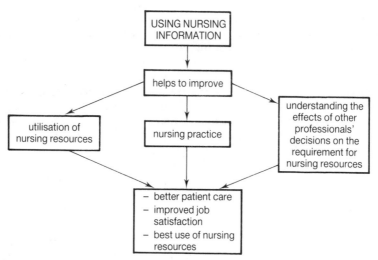

Fig. 6.9   Summary of benefits of using computerised nursing
information (National Health Service Management Executive,
1990b)

Choosing a Ward Nurse Management Information System (WNMIS)

Firstly there is a need to define exactly what the system is required to do. This can be done by providing a statement of Operational Requirements (OR) and then finding the system(s) which will provide this at an acceptable cost. The OR must reflect local requirements as no two sites will have exactly the same set up. A ward based system for 30 wards can cost between £80000 and £200000.

A guide to WNMIS currently available is produced by the NHS Resource Management Unit called *Nurse Management Systems a Guide to Existing and Potential Products*. (Greenhalgh and Company Limited, 1989) This guide gives a short description of the system, how it works, the standard reports it produces and a list of contacts and users. As new systems are introduced they will be included in the guide. There are more than 20 WNMIS available and already in use in some hospitals. These can be divided into the following:

Group A – those systems which deal primarily with patient information.
Group B – those which deal predominantly with nurse management information.
Group C – those which deal with both patient and nurse management information.

Examples of some of these systems are shown in Appendix 2.

District nursing information systems

The successful development and implementation of community computer systems, like hospital systems, depends on accurate and timely information. Since the patients are not being nursed in hospital, district nurses require a method of collecting data about patients in their homes, storing the data and being able to transfer data into a health care information system upon returning to base.

An example of an information system, designed for use in the community, is one based on the principle of a 'host' computer system. The host computer is fed by hand-held terminals issued to each of the staff working in the community. (Goldberg, 1987) The host system is a comprehensive community health package 'COMCARE' with which a hand-held Psion Organiser computer is used to collect the data. The two main inputs to the system are the patient registration, which creates the client index and opens episodes for each professional group currently treating the patient, and a daily activity log which is used by each member of staff to record information on the contacts with individual patients. Information on clinic and other activity is also recorded. The daily activity log allows staff to record attendance time and official mileage for payment and costing purposes.

The Psion computer has a RAM of 64k and takes two datapacks (EPROM chips) of up to 64k each. The datapacks, holding data collected by staff in the course of their work, can be taken or sent back to base, that is the host computer, to which the data can be transferred, stored and processed.

Occupational health information systems

There is increasing use of computer facilities throughout the whole health care system. Occupational health (OH) is no exception. In the workplace, systems are available for managing, analysing and reporting medical, health and safety, hazards and health physics data. Health and safety information could include personal and workplace sampling data, employee work and exposure histories, material safety, problem monitoring and incident information. Information on actual and potential hazards can facilitate compliance with hazard regulations, safety, labelling, emergency procedures and collection of COSHH data (Control of Substances Hazardous to Health). OH departments can have access to national databases such as the Health and Safety Executive (HSE) and Prestel, via a modem.

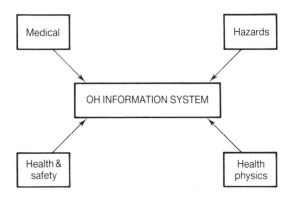

Fig. 6.10   An OH information system (A. Trueman, 1991)

Health physics information could be generated where special health surveillance is needed, for example, of those working with radiation. Information originating from dosimeters, bioassay and detection equipment can be analysed for regulatory compliance, dose management and reporting. Medical information could include a complete medical, work and exposure history for each employee, illness and injury details, lifestyle information and training details. Access to a database such as MASTA (Medical Advisory Service for Travellers Abroad) can provide information for employees who may be travelling to areas of particular risk, thus enabling appropriate vaccination to be given.

For nurses working in an OH department the primary function of the health care/personnel information system is to provide a record of information, to display and store information for a permanent record, and to print out information on records such as daily throughput, COSHH data, client recall dates, vaccination details and screening programmes. Sensitive information can be protected by the use of passwords or user identification (ID). The ID code would probably be changed monthly.

Outcome information

The final 'outputs' of hospitals are patients who have been discharged or who have died. Intermediate outputs include numbers of operations performed, diagnostic tests carried out, meals served, etc. Most outcome information is concerned with reporting on the efficiency of the service provided, and the efficient use of resources. Most measures of efficiency, that is input/output relationships, can be used as 'performance indicators'. Other measures of the use of resources, such as length of stay (LoS) can also be used.

Information on morbidity and mortality, patient throughput, waiting lists etc. will be available from HSIs. Critics of the use of HSIs may say that these indicators do not take sufficient account of 'outcomes', or quality of care. It is a reasonable assumption that improvements in efficiency should lead to improvements in effectiveness, or the quality of outcomes.

Effectiveness relates to the outcome in terms of the continuing physical and mental health of the patient/client population following episodes of care, *see* Fig. 6.11. It should be stressed that outcome information is usually obtained from quantitative data and does not necessarily, therefore, give information on the quality of the service provided. Some indication of quality can be obtained from qualitative outcome measures such as those discussed in the next chapter.

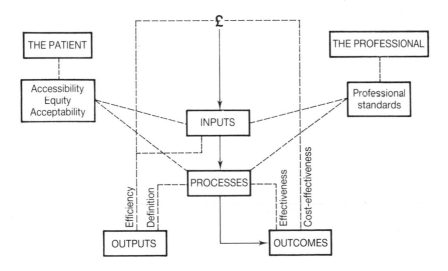

Fig. 6.11 Concepts of performance in health care (A. Trueman, 1991)

Datasets generated on a costed case basis, from the invoicing process, will enable detailed service use to be measured more accurately.

Health Service Indicators (HSIs)

The introduction of general management into the NHS heightened the need for management information. HSIs, which are statistics presented in a clear and systematic way, were developed and use existing sources of data set in a national perspective. Their aim is to help managers, clinicians and other professionals in providing more effective health services. HSIs enable managers to compare their own DHA's performance with that of other DHAs in England. Relevant questions can be raised about services they provide. In particular, instances of relatively low or high achievement can be easily identified. They do not, however, provide ready made answers.

Most of the indicators are simple ratios such as cost per case, nursing staff per occupied bed, deaths and discharges per available bed and provision per 1000 relevant population. HSIs are a tool for use by NHS managers at every level but are directed in the first instance at DHAs. They are not absolute measures of performance but give an idea of the service being provided. This enables pertinent questions to be asked with the objective of improving the provision of health care. The HSI package is distributed free to all RHAs and DHAs and contains over 400 indicators. The data are stored on floppy discs and are available for use with software such as Lotus Symphony and Lotus 1-2-3, to run on IBM compatible computers. There are only a handful of indicators of quality and outcome such as neo-natal mortality by weight. The vast majority are indicators of structure/input and process. Research into indicators of outcome may produce suitable outcome HSIs in the future, which give an indication of the quality of the service provided.

Data Protection Act 1983 (Parliament, 1984)

Computers are used throughout society to collect, store, process and distribute information. Much of this information is about people. The purpose of this Act is to protect individuals about whom information is held on computer. It does not cover information which is held and processed manually, for example, in ordinary paper files. Definitions within the Act include the following:

1. **Data** means information recorded in a form in which it can be processed by equipment operating automatically in response to instructions given for that purpose.
2. **Personal data** means data consisting of information which relates to a living individual who can be identified from that information (or from that or other data in the possession of the data user) including any expression of opinion about the individual but not any indication of the intentions of the data user in respect of that individual.
3. **Data subject** means the individual who is the subject of personal data.
4. **Data user** means a person who holds data.
5. **Computer bureau** means an organisation which processes personal data for Data Users or which allows Data Users to process data on their computers.
6. **Processing**, in relation to data, means amending, augmenting, deleting or re-arranging the data or extracting information constituting the data . . . in relation to the data subject. This shall not be construed as applying to any operation performed only for the purpose of preparing the text for documents i.e. word processing.
7. **Disclosing**, in relation to data, includes disclosing information extracted from the data. Where the identification of the individual, who is the subject of personal data, depends partly on the information constituting the (computer held) data, and partly on other information in the possession of the data user, the data shall not be regarded as disclosed or transferred.

There are three unconditional exemptions relating to personal data which:

(a) are required to be exempt for the purpose of safeguarding national security;
(b) the user is required by law to make public;
(c) is held by an individual and concerned only with the management of his personal, family or household affairs or held by him only for recreational purposes.

Every data user who holds personal data must, unless the data are exempt, be registered with the Data Protection Registrar.

Data protection principles

Registered Data Users must comply with the Data Protection Principles in relation to the personal data they hold. The Principles state that personal data shall:

(a)   be collected and processed fairly and lawfully;
(b)   be held only for the lawful purposes described in the register entry;
(c)   be used only for those purposes and only be disclosed to those people described in the register entry;
(d)   be adequate, relevant and not excessive in relation to the purpose for which they are held;
(e)   be accurate and, where necessary, kept up to date;
(f)   be held no longer than is necessary for the registered purpose;
(g)   be surrounded by proper security.

Subject access

An individual is entitled, on making a written request, to be supplied by any Data User with a copy of any personal data held about him or her. The Data User may make a charge for supplying this information. This right is called the 'subject access right'. This right does not always apply, for example, where giving subject access would be likely to prejudice the prevention or detection of crime.

Data protection and health care information systems

Much of the information in the health care field is held on computer, and much of this is personal data. This information would include that generated from the computerisation of health care and personnel records. This means that the NHS must comply with the Data Protection Act and must register as a data user and a computer bureau for three groups of data subjects:

  (i)   patients
 (ii)   staff
(iii)   other purposes

As far as security and access of information is concerned, personal information may be treated differently depending on the sensitivity of the information. As far as health care and personnel records are concerned this can be classified into three categories:

1.   **Registerable personal information** which would include information that is common knowledge such as names, home and work addresses, home and work telephone numbers, job titles, grades.
2.   **Confidential personal information** which includes named financial and medical information (as well as diagnostic and operation codes related to patient unit numbers).

3. **Secure personal information** which includes named information specified by the Data Protection Registrar as being particularly sensitive, for example:

(a) genetic, contraceptive, abortion and infertility services;
(b) racial origins, political/religious opinions, criminal convictions, sexual life and physical/mental health;
(c) persons suffering from mental illness, addiction and sexually transmitted diseases, including AIDS.

In general this information should not be printed, and distribution and access should be carefully controlled. User identification (ID) (passwords or codes) can be used to restrict access to information systems such as the PAS, PMI, occupational health and personnel.

Training needs

Nurses must acquire the knowledge and skills to enable them to maximise the opportunities presented to them both in the field of information technology, and the application of IT to health care, particularly to nursing. Knowledge and skills will include the following:

At ward level:

- operating a computer keyboard.
- operating nursing programs/systems (WNMIS, PMI and PAS).
- understanding dependency systems.
- patient care planning.

Additionally for more senior managers:

- management (of people and information).
- finance and budgeting.
- business principles.
- planning.

Since computers may replace all or part of a manual system, there need to be contingency plans in case the system goes down. How long can we manage if the system is out of use? What are the implications of having to revert to a manual system?

Data/program integrity, that is the quality, availability and accuracy of computerised data and programs needs to be maintained. Accidental or malicious alteration, loss or destruction, **sabotage (!!)** is always a possibility. This may, of course, occur as a result of hardware or software failure, or as a result of human error. There is always a risk that unauthorised users may get access to sensitive data, whether directly via terminals (networks) or by means of database query facilities (modem). This may lead to a breach of confidentiality or an intrusion of patient or staff privacy. User ID therefore must be carefully monitored and controlled.

Summary

This is an exciting time, with increasingly sophisticated computer systems providing the facility to collect, process, store and distribute a wealth of information. Not only the amount of information which is, and will be, available, but the type of information and the ways in which it can, and will be, both generated and presented.

The use of computerised information systems offers nurses, and other health care professionals, the opportunity to minimise the amount of paperwork involved in patient care, thus enabling them to spend more time with their patients. The availability of reliable and relevant information, to inform management decisions, should lead to better and more effective use of nursing and other health care resources. Figure 6.12 summarises the use of a ward based information system and its links with the hospital information system.

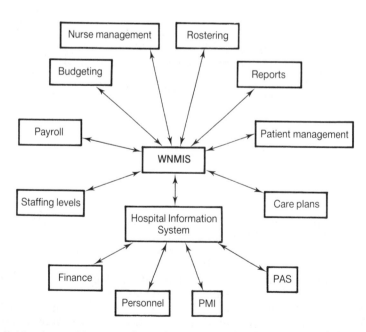

Fig. 6.12   A ward-based information system (A. Trueman, 1991)

Appendix 1

Operating Room Scheduling Office System (ORSOS)

A resource management system for use in operating theatres is available. This system is being used in a number of districts and provides sophisticated and comprehensive information/decision support for surgical resource management. The main features are:

1. Resource maintenance, database of staff, operating theatre suites, procedures performed, session times and preventative maintenance schedules.
2. Case scheduling, automatic appointment booking, collection of case data, printing of theatre lists, case records and theatre register and provision of daily management reports on utilisation and productivity.
3. Inventory control, which provides and stores information on surgeon preferences and procedures and can include actual and projected stock usage by surgeon and procedure. Charging details can be generated automatically as well as information on a costed case basis. The system can be interfaced with the hospital's supplies and finance systems. Bar coding can also be used.
4. Management reporting, which generates standard reports on topics such as volume statistics, utilisation of facilities, productivity of personnel, surgeon time per procedure, surgeon session utilisation and cost per DRG.

Appendix 2

The following are examples of Ward Nurse Management Information Systems (WNMIS) from each of the three groups referred to on page 157.

GROUP A – those systems which deal primarily with patient information.

EXELCARE (Price Waterhouse)

This system produces individual care plans based on locally determined standards. It uses this information to identify nursing resources required for each shift (to assist redeployment decisions), and to understand the cost of patient care related to these resources.

Criteria for care (Istel)

This system is designed to provide a means of identifying 'workload' and therefore the staff required, to enable their better deployment. By also recording information about actual staff on duty, it identifies variances.

Teamwork (North West Regional Health Authority)
Demand Methodology and Management Information System for Nursing

This system uses a methodology based on a formula (derived from research) to arrive at either prospective or retrospective hours required to provide a 'good' level of care. The formula uses a few simple workload indicators together with established coefficients to arrive at the hours required.

nCARE (L. McKendry)

This is a system designed to allow users to define ward based core care plans (using local standards/policies and procedures). These can then be called up and amended rather than drawn up from scratch. This system is currently available linked to the Financial Information Project (FIP) Ward Nursing System.

NMS (Design Management Systems)
Nurse Management System

This is a workload calculation system. It is designed to prospectively and retrospectively assess individual patient needs for staff time and to compare this to staff hours available. This is used for cost analysis, budgeting and planning.

GROUP B – those systems which deal predominantly with nurse management information

ANSOS – (Atwork Health Systems)
Automated Nurse Staffing Office System

This system provides a facility for drawing up staff rosters and recording staff hours worked for transfer to the payroll. There is an acuity/dependency facility, or the system can receive information from other systems and use this to compare staff required against staff available. The system costs the individual staff hours and, therefore, has the potential for reports for ward budgeting and financial management.

MERIT (Merit)
Nurse Deployment System

This is a nurse deployment system designed to produce rosters for staff and recording staff actual hours worked for transfer to the payroll. By costing these hours in great detail, a number of reports for ward budgeting and financial management are possible.

CRESTBOND (Crestbond)
Nurse Rostering System

This rostering system is aimed at speeding up the rostering process, as well as recording the hours worked and not worked by location for individual staff in sufficient detail for payroll requirements and costing. By costing the rostering process, it facilitates budgeting at ward level and monitors the use of resources.

SENS (South East Thames Regional Health Authority)
South East Nursing System

This is a workload calculation system based on patient dependency, either on a prospective or retrospective basis. A record of hours available is collected and compared, to assist in decisions to move staff to areas of greatest need.

Nurse manager (Whitehorse)

This system provides personnel records, a manual and automatic rostering function and timesheet information for payroll purposes. It also provides a care planning facility, and a workload measurement facility from either dependency or acuity, allowing for analyses of variance.

PCP – Nurse Management System (Priority Care Personnel)

This system is designed as a management system for the control of resources consumed by bank and agency staff, or any group of 'ad hoc' staff. By recording the actual hours worked of these staff the system provides both payroll reports and costing information for budgetary purposes.

NISCM – Nursing Information System for Change Management (J.D.M. Management Services)

This is available in both manual and computerised versions. It provides a method of calculating workload, either prospectively or retrospectively, and includes direct recording by nurses of 'what they do' which is used in understanding the workload as well as deriving it.

Group C – those systems which deal with both patient and nurse management information

FIP (General Automation/Istel/Siemens/South West Thames Regional Health Authority)

Financial Information Project – Ward Nursing System

This system identifies workload from a daily assessment of an individual patient's 'needs', and uses this with information about the staff available to redeploy staff as required. This information is then used operationally in the production of care plans. It can also produce a range of bed utilisation reports.

Sasha UK Ltd.
Ward Nursing System

This is a system comprising a number of modules run separately or as an integrated suite. These include: care planning, workload calculation (via care plan or acuity/dependency), rostering/timesheet and nursing manpower (nurse management) and costing.

TDS7000 (TDS Healthcare Systems Corporation)

This system is designed to computerise the administrative activities of the nurse, and from this to also provide information to manage the nursing resources. It provides patient registration and location tracking via the Patient Administration System (PAS), order entry and result reporting, clinical records (including drug administration) as well as nursing records and care plans. This system is currently used by some of the Resource Management Initiative (RMI) sites and is one of the few available systems with a fully integrated PAS. It can also be linked with a rostering system such as ANSOS.

CRESCENDO (CHC Software Care Ltd.)

This system's facilities include care planning, personnel, rostering, workload measurement, quality assurance, order entry, result reporting and electronic mail. A computer based training package is available with this system and covers an introduction to computing, an overview of the nursing process and CRESCENDO care planning.

Note Further details of these and other WNMIS can be found in *Nurse Management Systems: A Guide to Existing and Potential Products*, produced and updated 3 monthly by Greenhalgh and Company Limited.

List of abbreviations

BBS – Bulletin Board System
CBMS – Computer Based Messaging Systems
CD – Compact Disc
CMC – Computer Mediated Communication
COSHH – Control of Substances Hazardous to Health
CPU – Central Processing Unit
CSSD – Central Sterile Supply Department
DHA – District Health Authority
DIS – District Information System
DISS – District Information Support System
DoH – Department of Health
DRG – Diagnosis Related Group
EPROM – Erasable programmable Read Only Memory
FAX – Facsimile Machine
FHSA – Family Health Service Authority
FIP – Financial Information Project
FPC – Family Practitioner Committee
GP – General Practitioner

GPFH – General Practitioner Fund Holder
HSI – Health Service Indicator
HISS – Hospital Information Support Systems project
ID – Identification
IT – Information Technology
k – kilobyte
LAN – Local Area Network
mb – megabyte
MDS – Minimum Data Scts
MPI – Master Patient Index
MS-DOS – Microsoft – Disc Operating System
NHS – National Health Service
NHSME – National Health Service Management Executive
OPCS – Office of Population Censuses and Surveys
PAS – Patient Administration System
PC – Personal Computer
PMI – Patient Master Index
RAM – Random Access Memory
RHA – Regional Health Authority
RIS – Regional Information System

RM – Resource Management
RMI – Resource Management Initiative
ROM – Read Only Memory

VDU – Visual Display Unit
WAN – Wide Area Network
WNMIS – Ward Nurse Management Information System

Glossary of computing terms

Backup file is a copy of a file, held outside a computer system, to be used in the event of the original file being corrupted.

Bar-code reader is an input device used to scan a pattern of lines, using either optical or magnetic sensing techniques. The line pattern is coded information about the item to which it relates, for example, the price and description of an item in a shop or hospital stores.

Bit (BInary digiT) is one of the digits used in binary notation, i.e. 0 or 1. It is the smallest unit of storage by a computer.

Byte is a fixed number of bits, often corresponding to a single character, for example, a letter or a number.

CAL (Computer Assisted Learning) is the commonest of a number of terms describing uses of a computer in education and training.

Computer is a machine which, under the control of a stored program, automatically accepts and processes data, and supplies the results of that processing. (Mainframe, minicomputer and microcomputer.)

Computer graphics is the representation of information by a computer in graphical form, the display being either as charts or diagrams in hard copy or as animation on a visual display unit (VDU).

Cursor is a character that indicates the current display position on a visual display unit (VDU). On many devices it flashes on and off.

Database is a collection of structured data.

Data processing (DP) is the tradi-

tional name given to business information processing.

Data protection is the establishment of safeguards to preserve the integrity, privacy and security of data.

Data retrieval is the search for, or selection of, data from some areas of store linked to the computer.

Directory is a list of file names, together with information enabling the files to be retrieved from the backing store by the operating system.

Disc drive is the mechanism which causes the discs to rotate between read/write heads.

DOS is the common abbreviation for Disc Operating System, the portion of the operating system that deals with access to and management of files and programs stored on disc.

Electronic mail is the use of computer systems to transfer messages between users. It is usual for messages to be held in a central store, for retrieval at the recipient's convenience.

Electronic Pen is used to read hand written data.

Expert system is a computer system containing organised knowledge so that it can perform some of the functions of a human expert.

File is an organised collection of related records.

Floppy disc is a lightweight, flexible magnetic disc which behaves as if rigid when rotated rapidly. Also called a diskette.

Gigobyte is approximately one hundred million bytes.

Hard copy is computer output printed on paper (a printout).

Hard disc is a rigid magnetic disc. It normally allows a higher recording density than a floppy disc, thus providing more storage for the same physical dimensions.

Hardware is the name given to the physical components of a computer system, including peripherals such as keyboard, screen and printer.

Information technology (IT) is the distribution and use of information by means of computers and telecommunications networks.

Input device is a peripheral unit which can accept data, presented in the appropriate machine readable form, decode it and transmit it as electrical impulses to the central processing unit (CPU).

Interface is the hardware and software required to connect two devices in a computer system.

Keyboard on a computer is usually QWERTY – laid out in the standard keyboard pattern, or numeric – one with only numbers.

Kilobyte is 1024 bytes (characters or letters).

Log in/log out is the correct method by which a remote terminal user enters or disconnects from a multi-access system.

Megabyte is approximately one million bytes.

Menu is one of a series of option choices displayed to lead the user through the stages of an interactive program.

Microchip consists of a sliver of silicon on which many thousands of transistors are etched. There are different chips for different functions.

Microprocessor is a single chip that performs the functions of a central processing unit.

Modem (modulator/demodulator) is a device to allow conversion of bits into analog electrical impulses for transmission over telephone-type circuits, and vice versa.

Mouse is an input device which the user moves around on a flat surface thereby causing a cursor to move around the display screen (VDU).

Network is a linked set of computer systems, sometimes widely dispersed geographically, capable of sharing computing power or storage facilities.

Output device is a peripheral unit which translates signals from the computer into human-readable form or into a form suitable for reprocessing by the computer at a later stage.

Password (ID) is a sequence of characters which must be presented to a computer system before it will allow access to the system or parts of the system, e.g., a particular file. Passwords are used for security reasons.

Printer is an output device producing characters or graphic symbols on paper. Examples are daisy-wheel, dot-matrix, golf-ball, ink-jet and laser printers.

RAM (Random Access Memory) is computer memory which may be read from and written to by the programmer.

ROM (Read Only Memory) is computer memory which may not be written to by the programmer. The software in the ROM is fixed during manufacture.

Scanner is an electronic reader which converts printed text and graphics into code for input into the computer for use with other applications.

Software is the name given to programs, routines, procedures and their associated documentation which can be used on a computer system.

Speech synthesizer is an output device that generates sound similar to human speech on receipt of digital signals.

Terminal is the term used to describe any input/output device which is used to communicate with the computer from a remote site.

Touch screen is an input device which allows menu choices by touching the VDU.

Visual Display Unit (VDU) is a terminal device, incorporating a cathode ray tube (like a television set), on which text can be displayed. It is usually used in conjunction with a keyboard.

A Glossary of other useful terms

Accountability is the obligation to render account or report on one's performance.

Acuity is a (nurse) workload measure.

Budget is a plan formulated as monetary authorisation of allowable cost or expenditure.

Budgeting is the process of preparing budgets through which desired workloads/outputs are balanced with the costs of resources/inputs.

Case mix costing involves the recording of information about patients which will allow them to be classified by diagnostic characteristics, treatments, etc., *see* DRGs.

Diagnosis related groups (DRGs) is the name of a system of classifying acute, non-psychiatric inpatients according to their diagnostic characteristics and related health care resource requirements.

Effectiveness is concerned with outcomes rather than with routine inputs, and is concerned with the quality or benefit of outcomes.

Efficiency is concerned with improving the performance relationship between inputs of resources consumed and outputs of workload accomplished.

Episode of care refers to all the care received by a patient from first referral to outcome, for an episode of illness.

General management refers to the concept that managers should be committed to the efficiency and effectiveness of the total organisation and its goals rather than to the interests of individual functions or professions.

Management budgeting refers to the introduction of clinicians as budget holders together with clarifying individual manager's responsibilities and increasing accountability by agreeing targets and performance levels. This was one of the recommendations of the Griffiths Inquiry Report.

Minimum data set refers to the minimum amount of data which need to be collected to meet the Körner requirements.

Resource management can be defined as the efficient and effective use of assets, as measured in procedures, time and cost to accomplish one's objectives.

References

Cox, H. C., Harsanyi, B. and Dean, L. C. (1987). *Computers and Nursing: Application to Practice, Education and Research*. Prentice-Hall International, London.

Department of Health. (1989). *Working for Patients*. HMSO, London.

Evans, D. W. (1990). *People, Communication and Organisations.* 2nd. edn. Pitman, London.

Goldberg, B. and Savill, A. (1987). COMCARE on hand-held. *British Journal of Healthcare Computing*, **4(3)**, 23–5.

Greenhalgh and Company Limited (1990). *Nurse Management Systems: a Guide to Existing and Potential Products.* GCL, Macclesfield.

Koch, B. and Rankin, J. (Eds.), (1987). *Computers and Their Application In Nursing.* Harper and Row, London.

National Health Service Information Management Group and Department of Health. (1990). *Framework for Information Systems: The Next Steps.* HMSO, London.

National Health Service and Department of Health and Social Security Steering Group on Health Services Information. (1982). *A Report from working group E: Manpower Information.* DHSS, London. (Chairman: E. Körner).

National Health Service and Department of Health and Social Security Steering Group on Health Services Information. (1984). *Sixth Report: a Report on the Collection and Use of Financial Information in the National Health Service.* HMSO, London. (Chairman: E. Körner).

National Health Service Management Executive (1990a). *Personnel Issues.* NHSME, London.

National Health Service Management Executive. (1990b). *Nursing Information Requirements: Identification and Computerisation.* NHSME, London.

NHS Management Inquiry Team. (1983). *NHS Management Inquiry. (Letter to the Secretary of State for Social Services.* The Team, London. (Team Leader: E. R. Griffiths).

Parliament. (1984). *Data Protection Act.* HMSO, London.

Perrin, J. (1990). *Resource Management in the NHS.* Chapman Hall, London.

Rathwell, T. (1987). *Strategic Planning in the Health Sector.* Croom Helm, Beckenham.

Willis, A. and Stewart, T. (1989). *Computers: a Guide to Choosing and Using.* Oxford University Press, Oxford.

Willis, L. D. and Linwood, M. E. (Eds.), (1984). *Measuring the Quality of Care.* Churchill Livingstone, Edinburgh.

Suggested Further Reading

Bakewell, K. G. B. (1984). *How to Organise Information.* Gower, London.

Bevan, G., Copeman, H., Perrin, J. and Rosser, R. (1980). *Health Care: Priorities and Management.* Croom Helm, Beckenham.

Brooks, R. (Ed.), (1986). *Management Budgeting in the NHS*. Health Services Manpower Review, Keele.

Department of Health and Social Security. (1985). *Management Budgeting*. DHSS, London. (HN(85)3).

Department of Health and Social Security (1986). *Resource Management (Management Budgeting) in Health and Authorities*. DHSS, London. (HC(86)34).

Handy, C. B. (1985). *Understanding Organisations*. 3rd edn. Penguin, Harmondsworth.

Hannagan, T. J. (1982). *Mastering Statistics*. Macmillan, London.

Harper, W. M. (1982). *Statistics*. 4th edn. Macdonald and Evans, Plymouth.

Holye, K. and Whitehead, G. (1979). *Business Statistics and Accounting Made Simple*. W. H. Allen, London.

Institute of Health Services Management. (1986). *Information Technology in Health Care – a Handbook*. IHSM/Kluwer, London.

King's Fund Centre. (1990). *Step by Step Guide to the Choosing of a Nurse Management System*. KFC, London.

Koch, H. C. H. (Ed.), (1988). *General Management in the Health Service*. Croom Helm, London.

Lewis, C. D. (1984). *Managing with Micros: Management Uses of Microcomputers*. 2nd edn. Blackwell, Oxford.

National Health Service Training Authority. (1990). *Guide to the Implementation of Nursing Information Systems*. NHSTA, Bristol.

Sweeney, M. A. (1985). *The Nurse's Guide to Computers*. Macmillan, New York.

7 Quality assurance: the pathway to excellence

Introduction

Quality is the concern of everyone who provides a service and everyone who uses that service (Keighley, 1989). This belief is the central ethos of 'Total Quality Management', it is also one that underpins the National Health Service (NHS) reforms conveyed in the White Paper, Working for Patients (Department of Health, 1989a), where purchasers and providers will negotiate contracts, agree what constitutes quality and operationalise this agreement through standards that are explicit, observable and measurable.

This view of quality has entered the arena of health care following exposure to similar movements promoted elsewhere by the following groups:

1. British industry, as reflected by British Standard 5750, 'quality systems' (British Standards Institute, 1987) a comprehensive three-part standard concerned with the establishment of comprehensive quality assurance systems throughout service and industrial sectors.
2. American management protagonists illustrated by the works *In Search of Excellence* (Peters and Waterman, 1982), and *A Passion for Excellence* (Peters and Austin, 1985).
3. Japanese industrial practices reflected in approaches such as Total Quality Management, Quality Circles and the moto, 'first we make people and then we make things.' (Keighley, 1989).

Alongside these practices from outside the domain of health care, there are also the influences from within, such as increasing consumerism as reflected by the development of 'consumer-orientated philosophies' (Newcomb and Kleiner, 1989); a strategy for nursing identified by the Department of Health outlining goals for standard setting, quality assessment and quality assurance (Department of Health, 1989b); various World Health Organization publications (cited by Healy, 1988); and also the American health care system. The latter has unfortunately been heavily influenced by negative factors such as the fear of lawsuits and the denial of accreditation, with therefore a subsequent loss of revenue. (Brenner, 1985). Brenner recognised at that time that Britain had an opportunity of developing quality assurance not because it had to but because it wanted to. This is therefore a different motivation to that experienced by the Americans and is one which is more akin to the values of Total Quality Management. However, since 1985 similar external pressures have also been experienced in the United Kingdom as a result of reorganisation of the NHS and subsequent legislation.

The motivation underpinning this chapter however relates more to the voluntary desire to make explicit the exact nature of the service that nursing is providing to the consumer. Nursing needs to undertake this task willingly if it is to consider itself to be a profession, criteria for which not only includes responsibility for setting, monitoring and maintaining its own standards and service, but also accountability to consumers for the service it seeks to provide.

Historically nursing's first experience with quality assurance is well recognised as being in the time of Florence Nightingale (Van Maanen, 1979; Lang and Clinton, 1984a). Nursing was seen by Nightingale (1859) as 'putting the patient in the best environment for nature to act upon him'. These values are therefore reflected in the standards that were important to Nightingale, particularly in relation to the environment. Such standards were concerned for example with the proximity of beds from windows, the thickness of mattresses, nutrition and fresh air. So what relevance do these influences have for health care today, in particular nursing, and how do they relate to the title of this chapter?

Certainly, as the largest workforce involved in healthcare, nursing and midwifery personnel comprise the most costly staffing component of the NHS, and will therefore increasingly be open to scrutiny in terms of its purpose and worth (Wilson and McNulty, 1991). However, even more important issues for nursing relate to the following essential questions:

What is nursing?
What is nursing's purpose?

Until nursing can answer these questions and until the values underpinning the answers can be made more explicit, it will not be possible to comprehensively specify what good nursing is, let alone what excellence in nursing is, and subsequently if the domain of nursing remains vague then it will also be impossible to assure a specific service to the consumer. This chapter aims to explore the pathways on which to embark when striving for excellence in whatever nursing is finally considered to be.

Quality, institutions and purpose

According to Donabedian there are two major objectives that every institution concerned with health care and each practitioner within such institutions need to strive for. These are:

1. 'To provide care of the highest possible quality'
2. 'To provide that care at the lowest possible cost'

(Donabedian, 1989)

Donabedian considers these objectives to be inseparable, because poor care can result in harm. Such care is therefore wasteful, and wasteful care depletes the energies and resources which could have been used to benefit patients and clients. This sentiment is further reflected in Morris's (1989) view:

'Quality does cost money but so does the lack of it, and often the lack costs even more'

Keighley (1989) parallels this view with Ison's Law of Ten which states 'that it costs ten times less to identify and correct problems at the previous station of control than to leave the error to the next occasion it is possible to change the process'.

In human terms the cost of not getting things right is identified by Orlando (1961) in her study of nursing entitled the *Dynamic Nurse–Patient relationship*. Orlando differentiates between 'deliberate' and 'automatic' nursing actions in relation to patients' distress. Automatic actions by the nurse are ritualistic and do not attempt to validate the patients perceptions and cause of their distress. Ultimately such automatic actions, she suggests, causes the patient further harm. Deliberate actions, in contrast, are those responses by the nurse aimed at validating the cause of distress through interaction with the client, the positive outcome following such intervention being reduced distress.

This chapter having touched briefly on the background to quality assurance will now continue by exploring the terminology first, before then focussing predominantly on the process of quality assurance using Lang's quality assurance model as a structural framework. The chapter will then culminate in a presentation of one model designed for unit based care settings and conclude by re-visiting the concept of Total Quality Management briefly mentioned in the introduction.

Terminology

Jargon is widespread, terms numerous, and according to Healy (1988) 'semantics can lead to confusion'. Healy identifies a large number of terms used as part of health care quality assurance terminology internationally. He tries to introduce some order by classifying them into the four groups identified in Table 7.1.

Table 7.1   A classification of quality assurance terms (Healy 1988) with some examples of terms included in each category

Classification Group	Examples of terms
1. General and basic terms and concepts	EFFICIENCY EFFECTIVENESS PURCHASER QUALITY QUALITY ASSURANCE OUTCOME PROCESS STRUCTURE
2. Operational terms in management, design, process, certification, deficiencies, reliability, availability.	AUDIT CLINICAL REVIEW CRITERIA STANDARD MONITORING
3. Safety/risk	HAZARD RISK SAFETY
4. Economics	COST-BENEFIT ANALYSIS PREVENTION COSTS

Healy's paper is a comprehensive and in-depth study for those readers wishing to pursue a deeper understanding of the terminology. However just 'quality' and 'quality assurance', terms essential to the understanding and implementation of quality assurance practices in health settings will now be considered. Other terms important to the subject will be defined as they occur.

Quality is an abstract concept which is difficult to define precisely although many people have attempted this onerous task. In relation to health care and nursing, what is a quality service? Shaw (1986) considers that 'definitions of "quality" and related words are too elusive to merit the time of practical people.' However, Healy (1988) links the use of the word 'quality' to the following two senses:

1. The 'comparative sense' or 'degree of excellence'.

The key concepts here relate to ranking on a relative basis. Within nursing both Lang's and Van Maanen's definition of quality can be seen to include these aspects:

> 'quality is the process for the attainments of the highest *degree of excellence* in the delivery of patient or client care.'
>
> (Lang, 1976)

> 'quality is the *margin between* desirability and reality'
>
> (Van Maanen, 1981)

2. The 'fitness for purpose sense.'

The key concept here relates to the ability of a service to satisfy a particular need, in other words its appropriateness and effectiveness.

In nursing the latter sense is an essential area for development, in particular the relationship between purpose/outcome, nursing actions, and resources. The need for process-outcome and structure-process-outcome research in this area has been particularly highlighted by various writers. (Hamric, 1989; Lang and Clinton, 1984b; Watkins, 1990)

Further insights into the nature of quality are provided by Donabedian (1989) who considers that there are essentially three components:

1. The quality of technical care.
2. The goodness of the interpersonal relationship.
3. The goodness of the amenities of care.

He also suggests two other pre-conditions, these being access to care, and money. However Shaw (1986) considers quality to be primarily concerned with consumer satisfaction, although he also states it to be more than this by citing six further elements derived in part from Maxwell's (1984) work. These elements are appropriateness, equity, accessibility, effectiveness, acceptability and efficiency. Shaw considers 'appropriateness to be the key component' and this is also supported by Healy (1988) in terms of the 'fitness for purpose' previously identified. These six elements are defined in Table 7.2 where they are related to examples and questions relevant to nursing.

It is probably appropriate at this point to differentiate quality from quantity, as their differences mirror similar differences between the terms efficiency and effectiveness, and outputs and outcomes. In fact separating out these words into two separate clusters (Table 7.3) may help to isolate their differences.

In the past there has been confusion between the concepts of quality

Table 7.2 Definitions of the six key elements to quality summarised by Shaw (1986) but derived from Maxwell's work (1984), with also relevant examples and questions in nursing

Element	Definition	An example of relevance to nursing
Appropriateness	The service/procedure administered is one that the population/individual actually needs.	Expecting independent patients to get undressed and to wander around in nightclothes for one/two days prior to elective surgery/investigations may be inappropriate.
Equity	An equal share for everyone.	Are all people with terminal cancer at home given the opportunity of using the Macmillan (or similar) Nursing service?
Accessibility	The ease with which services are available. Constraints such as prohibitive distances, excessive waiting time, knowledge of the existence of a service, or other factors that may hinder access.	Through ignorance of care-givers about the existence of specific support groups, patients may be denied access to them.
Effectiveness	The extent to which an intended benefit has been achieved.	To what extent does tepid sponging reduce core temperatures or provide comfort to a patient? What is the effectiveness of this practice?

To what extent does health promotion change practice in relation to smoking or the transmission of the Human Immunodeficiency Virus (HIV)? |
| Acceptability | The extent to which the 'reasonable expectations' (Shaw 1986) of the consumer are satisfied. | What are the expectations of consumers in relation to care? How can we know if expectations are met if we do not know what they are? |

Table 7.2 *Continued*

Element	Definition	An example of relevance to nursing
		Campbell, et al (1985) identify the need to consider patients expectations when trying to model the patients world. Understanding the world through the client's eyes is central to interaction and interpersonal based nursing models e.g. Orlando (1961), Riehl-Sisca (1989), and Peplau (1952).
Efficiency	Relates benefits/outputs achieved to resources consumed i.e. physical, human, time, money. 'The greatest possible number of outputs for the least number of inputs' (Wilson & McAnulty 1991). Efficiency is increased if the number of outputs are increased for the same number of inputs, or alternatively if outputs are maintained but inputs reduced.	Is taking temperatures using electronic thermometers with disposable sensors more efficient in terms of nurses' time and the cost of equipment, than taking temperatures with mercury thermometers which have to remain in position for at least 8 minutes (Baker et al 1984) and also require cleaning?

Table 7.3 Quantity v Quality; related words are clustered according to their affiliation to these terms

Quantity	Quality
Efficiency	Effectiveness
Output	Outcome
Throughout	
Input	

and quantity particularly when the DHSS performance indicators, now named 'Health Service Indicators' (HSI), were initially introduced. HSIs are indicators of efficiency not effectiveness, providing information on outputs, throughputs and inputs rather than outcomes. **Outputs** are concerned with numbers (Perrin, 1990); for example the number of people discharged, and the number of patients cared for, whereas **outcomes** relate to the quality of these outputs (Perrin, 1990), that is the benefits. For example, whether patient dependency and the quality of life is improved as a result of treatments/operations; whether patients feel cared for, whether they feel respected as individuals, and whether they are satisfied with the care they receive, to name but a few. Outcomes are therefore more akin to the concept of effectiveness, whereas outputs (inputs and throughput) relate to efficiency.

Donabedian's model for the evaluation of quality of health care

Donabedian (1966), an American public health doctor whose model has been used world-wide states that the factors which influence the quality of health care may be simply divided into three groups. It was he who coined the terms **'structure'**, **'process'** and **'outcome'**. These terms, their definitions, other synonyms and examples are presented in Table 7.4.

Table 7.4   Donabedian's Structure, Process, and Outcome defined, with synonyms and examples

	Structure	**Process**	**Outcome**
Synonyms:	Inputs Resources	Throughputs Actions Content of care	Outputs Results
Definitions:	The setting in which care takes place.	The care given by health care professionals.	The results of structure and process combined.
Examples:	Resources Staff Equipment Education/training Heating/lighting	Assessment Planning Implementation Evaluation Knowledge	Health status Infection rates Immunization take-up rates Patient satisfaction Re-admission rates

Structure, process and outcome according to Donabedian are interlinked. In the past much greater emphasis was placed on the structural components of care and their relationship to health, particularly in nursing. Nightingale is exemplary in this view; her values about nursing centred around her beliefs about the role of the environment in recovery from illness. This concern for the environment and its relationship with nursing actions and outcome is now an explicit component of all nursing models today (Fawcett, 1984). However from our experiences we know that the lack of resources can affect the outcome of care. For example if no pressure regulating beds are available then the care of patients with pressure sores will be influenced negatively in the absence of sufficient numbers of staff to turn patients. Likewise the absence of supplies for mouthcare, eyecare packs and incontinence sheets severely limits the quality of care that can be given and subsequently the outcomes of that care may be affected. Although quantities of resources in these examples may influence the care that can be given it is important that optimal resources are considered in terms of cost-effectiveness. For example the more money that is spent per capita of the population in formal health care does not mean that health outcomes are improved, as demonstrated by comparing countries in Europe (Open University, 1985). Likewise having a large number of nurses on duty does not automatically result in higher quality care. This many of us have experienced when due to a 'fluke' on the off-duty more nurses than usual arrive; everyone else automatically thinks that the other person is doing a specific job and as a result many jobs get left undone!

The relationship between our actions and the outcomes of care we generally consider to be linked. This is however an assumption, as the outcome is not always related directly to the quality of care given or the process used (Wright, 1984), although correlation between the process of giving care and those of the outcome of care is something that requires considerably more research (Hamric, 1989). The difficulty of process-outcome research in nursing has been well recognised (Bloch, 1980). Some well known nursing studies have demonstrated a link between process and outcome, (e.g., those listed in Table 7.5) but much more work needs to be done on first identifying nursing concepts and explaining the relationships between them before the stage can be reached of prescribing actions where outcomes can be predicted with any degree of certainty. (Dickoff and James, 1968; Manley, 1991a).

Quality assurance in its literal sense means to 'guarantee' or 'assure' quality nursing care (Lang and Clinton, 1984a); but before quality can be assured, controlled or improved it must first be capable of being evaluated (British Standard Institute, 1979). However the most common meaning attributed to the term quality assurance relates to the all embracing process involved in attaining quality. This process involves converting values and beliefs into explicit standards, then measuring, monitoring, maintaining and reviewing these standards. In fact Lang's definition of quality identified earlier could more appropriately be

Table 7.5 Selected nursing research which relates nursing actions to outcome

Nurse Researcher	Nursing action	Outcomes
Haywood, J. (1975)	Information given pre-operatively	Post-operatively: Anxiety reduced Pain reduced Analgesic consumption reduced
Miller, A. (1985)	Using the nursing process with elderly care patients resident in institutions for longer than one month	Patient dependency reduced

considered a definition of quality assurance. Quality assurance as a process then can be represented by various models which describe what quality assurance is and identify its various components. Understanding the terms is essential so that nurses can contribute in a meaningful way at every level of health care in terms of quality assurance. The purpose of quality assurance is therefore 'to assure the consumer of nursing of a specified degree of excellence through continuous measurement and evaluation' (Schmadl, 1979).

Lang's quality assurance model

Lang's quality assurance model (1976) adapted by the American Nurses Association (1982), and Donabedian's evaluation model (1966) are two key works to understand when considering quality assurance not only with regards to nursing but for every area of health care provision. The American Nurses Association model has been further simplified by Kitson and Kendall (1986) into the three fundamental stages of:

1. Describing and setting objectives.
2. Measuring and monitoring.
3. Taking action.

These three stages form the key areas of focus in the Dynamic Standard Setting System (DySSSy) developed by the Royal College of Nursing's (RCN) Standards of Care Project (Royal College of Nursing, 1990). Each of the three macro-stages subsuming the steps from the original model. These steps are arranged in the cyclical relationship illustrated in Fig. 7.1.

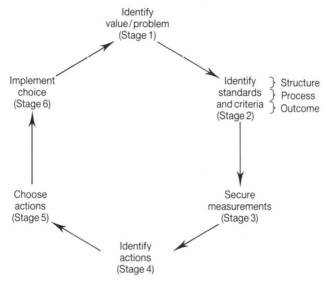

Fig. 7.1   The American Nurses Association's model of quality
assurance (1982), adapted from Lang's model (1976)

This model is a dynamic model as the values present in Stage 1 will be influenced by changing trends and developments within the profession, society and technology. For example there are changes in the emphasis, focus and purpose of nursing today compared with those 30–40 years ago when concepts such as 'self-care', 'patient-participation', 'mutual goal setting' and 'nursing diagnosis' were unknown within British nursing. Similarly changes within society and technology will alter our values; for example a greater awareness and responsibility for factors affecting one's health as a result of media coverage which alter our expectations. Computerisation and sophisticated equipment now makes possible options which were previously impossible. Hence, identifying and agreeing the area of common ground in terms of values is for this author an important starting point on the path towards excellence.

Establishing philosophical values and beliefs

Our behaviour is greatly influenced by our beliefs and values (Lancaster and Lancaster, 1982; Fitzpatrick, 1989). Our values in turn are also affected by our personal and professional beliefs and scientific knowledge (Lang, 1976) (*see* Chapter 2). When working within a team, be that a team of nurses or the multi-disciplinary team, identifying values and beliefs can form the foundation of the team's direction, aims and objectives. Common aims and objectives shared by the whole team are a powerful contribution to working cohesively and with common purpose. These beliefs together with our values and attitudes can be made explicit through a statement of philosophy and purpose. Such a statement can help when difficult decisions have to be made, by providing direction. A statement of values and beliefs can identify incongruences in practice; for example, if a group of nurses share the view that their purpose is to help patients become self-caring within their potential to do so then it would be incongruent practice to prevent patients and relatives from making their own tea and coffee within an institutional setting if they so wished. A team philosophy can never reflect everyone's values and beliefs about everything, but it can identify areas of common ground and agreement about the nature and purpose of nursing and/or the multidisciplinary team. One method used by a team of intensive care nurses together with physiotherapists and the unit's technician in developing a philosophy was to combine two processes simultaneously (Warfield and Manley, 1990); a value clarification exercise combined with a nominal group technique. The value clarification exercise used centred on the following aspects:

(a)   the purpose of the service.
(b)   the four concepts (the metaparadigm of nursing) central to all nursing models (Fawcett 1984) thus reflecting the domain and concern of nursing, these are the nature of:

  (*i*)   Nursing.
 (*ii*)   The individual person.
(*iii*)   Health.
(*iv*)   The environment of care/society.

(see Chapter 5)

(c)   how individuals learn, as this particular area was used as a learning environment for post-registration students; additionally the personal learning and development of all staff was valued by both staff and clinical management.
(d)   the attributes of a good team, nursing and multi-disciplinary.

The value clarification exercise used is outlined in Table 7.6, and although the example refers to an intensive therapy unit (ITU), little modification would be required for its use elsewhere.

The nominal group technique (Delbecq, Van der Ven, and Gust-afson, 1975) is a technique which allows everyone's values to be collected and built up over time, as it is never possible for all staff to meet at once. The value clarification exercise is therefore carried out in small groups depending on who is available until everyone has parti-cipated. All values and beliefs stated are therefore carried through to the final statement. The total approach used is outlined in Table 7.7.

Table 7.6 The value clarification exercise used by Warfield and Manley (1990) as the basis of writing a philosophy in an intensive therapy unit (ITU).

I believe the purpose of ITU is . . .
I believe my purpose in ITU is . . .
I believe critically ill patients need . . .
If I was a patient in ITU I would like . . .
I believe families/relatives/significant others of ITU patients value . . .
I believe I can help an ITU patient . . .
As a member of the ITU team I feel valued when . . .
I believe the ITU environment for staff should be . . .
I believe the ITU environment for patients should be . . .
I believe individuals learn best when . . .
What beliefs do you hold about the nurse-patient relationship?
What do you value most highly as an ITU member?
What do you believe makes a good team?
Other values and beliefs I consider important are . . .

Table 7.7 One approach to gathering staff values and beliefs using a nominal group technique (Manley 1990)

1. Identification of staff with previous experience of using or writing a philosophy.
2. Explanation and clarification of philosophy, values and beliefs, its purpose and why it is important.
3. Groups of approximately four persons brainstorm their beliefs and values in relation to the value clarification exercise.
4. One person from each group documents the brainstorming exercise and represents the group's views.
5. Points identified by other groups are added to the points made by the first group, if not already identified.
6. This is continued until every member of staff has been provided with an opportunity of participating.
7. The result is a random collection of values and beliefs reflecting the whole staff's values and beliefs.
8. Using a wordprocessor (it would be extremely time consuming and arduous task without one!) the words reflecting similar values and beliefs are grouped together through 'cutting and pasting' (*see* Chapter 6)
9. Sentences can then be compiled using the words grouped.
10. The order of the sentences are then arranged stating purpose first, followed by paragraphs which flow in their content from broad to specific. This, the first draft, is then circulated to all staff for comment.
11. The final draft once completed can be shared with patients and relatives and other professional colleagues, provision having been made for revision and updating.

As new staff come and go, and as new problems test the beliefs held, the philosophy if it is to be dynamic will need to reflect such changes. Revision of a philosophy may be necessary for the following reasons:

1. New staff introduced to the philosophy in their orientation may bring with them new ideas for discussion.
2. Through caring for patients and relatives issues may be raised which need to be discussed and assimilated within the philosophy.
3. Regular periodic review.
4. The philosophy may not be helpful with particular difficult decisions and so further refinement and clarification may be required.
5. The values stated may be unrealistic and impossible to achieve, and with experience of trying to operationalise them may require changing.
6. Changes in society itself may mean that values and beliefs need revisiting.

Although this approach allows a unit philosophy to result which subsequently will guide the standards written, there may exist other priority problems or areas of concern which need to be addressed as a matter of urgency. In some circumstances then it may be more important to identify the values relating to a single problem, then resolving that problem before returning to the philosophy at a later date. Lang's quality assurance model (1976) can therefore be employed at both macro- and micro- levels when striving for the provision of better services. Regardless of which values are focussed on first, it is the application of them to practice which is an important second step. No statement of values however good will be of any value unless operationalised.

Values once identified can be operationalised by converting them to general objectives from which specific objectives or standards can then be derived (Table 7.8). The type of standards derived in Fig. 7.8 include examples of process standards. These are concerned with actions relating to what nurses do in respect of the roles of clinician, educator and manager. An alternative term to process standard is 'performance standard'. Performance standards are very valuable as a basis of Individual Performance Review (IPR), as they explicitly state what is expected from staff and will be referred to again later.

Further illustrations of how values influence behaviour can be seen in models of nursing. Nursing models represent what nursing is from the perspective of specific nurse theorists. (*see* Chapter 5). The values held by the nurse theorist will be reflected in the model and will influence the stated purpose and role of nursing. For example central values in Orem's model (1985) are to do with an individual's ability to be self-caring. The purpose of nursing would therefore be to assist the

Table 7.8   How stated values may be operationalised. (Warfield and Manley, 1990)

Stated value	General objective	Specific objective (example)
Families/relatives/ significant others are important people to patients.	To involve relatives in care to the extent they and the patient wish involvement. (clinical)	All relatives are asked about their expectations of care.
All staff can grow and develop as individuals. Such personal growth increases job satisfaction and benefits patients.	All staff are helped to identify their personal and professional needs and to select appropriate methods to develop them. (educational)	Individuals with perceptors negotiate individual learning contracts.
Individuals work best within a team which shares common values.	Values and beliefs are explicit when recruiting new staff so as to attract people of similar philosophy. (managerial)	Every applicant is issued with a unit philosophy.

patient/client to become as self-caring as possible. In contrast, Roy (1984) considers that health relates to an individual's ability to adapt to internal and external stimuli. The purpose of nursing therefore is to help the individual

(a)   to develop and enhance coping strategies for responding to stimuli.
(b)   to help reduce the stimuli impinging on the individual.

Rogers (1989) also views the nature of the person from a very different perspective; in no way can the individual be understood by reducing them into parts (even bio-psychosocial parts!), they can only be understood as energy fields coextensive with the environment. Rogers sees human beings as becoming more complex in their evolution and therefore explains insomnia in elderly people and hyperactivity in children as due to this increasing complexity. Whatever one may think of Rogers ideas there is one thing that this viewpoint clearly demonstrates and that is the major influence that our values have on our attitudes and behaviour. From Rogers' perspective the view that elderly people cannot sleep because they are becoming more complex results in a much more positive perspective on old age, than the view that old age is about increasing degeneration and disability.

Table 7.9   Response to influence (after Kelman, 1958) (cited by Handy, 1985).

Response	Definition	Associated management style	Examples
Comply	Do as directed by others	Autocratic, one-way communication. No consultation or participation. Rules and regulations ensure change is implemented and the influence is maintained.	Commonly used examples include the way that the nursing process was implemented initially. An alternative mandate is reflected in the view that 'primary nursing will be implemented'.
Identify	Identifying with the source of influence or the rationale behind the ideas being introduced.	Charismatic leadership style. Two way communication – consultative more than participative. Positive feedback and recognition required to maintain the influence.	The innovative and charismatic ward sister who after achieving great change then leaves. The staff remaining then revert back to previous ways of operating.
Internalise	Owning ideas as if they were one's own.	Participative, democratic leadership style. Management which is open, trusting and encourages and supports personal development. Individuals are empowered to take risks and to try new and creative ideas.	Change is successfully achieved and maintained. Staff are self-directing and self motivating.

When choosing a nursing model, or part of a model, for the purpose of guiding care then it is first necessary to have considered closely one's values and beliefs before selecting a model which is then hopefully congruent with these values. If one is operating within a system where values are congruent then it is more likely that ideas have been internalised and owned and individuals are self-directing and self motivating. Support for this view can be seen in the work of Kelman (1958) (cited by Handy, 1985) who suggests that we respond to influences in three ways; by compliance and identification with, or internalisation of ideas presented to us. An analysis of these three types are illustrated in Table 7.9.

Why is it important to be aware of Kelman's work in relation to quality assurance one may ask?

Firstly if staff have been involved and have participated actively in identifying values and in quality assurance, then they are more likely to have internalised ideas and therefore will be self-directing. If, on the other hand, staff have been told to implement a quality assurance system without consultation and participation then it is likely that they may only comply with the change, not necessarily willingly or cooperatively. Related to Kelman's work are the approaches to change commonly described as 'bottom up' and 'top down'. 'Top-down' methods tend to require staff complying with ideas rather than owning them. Whereas 'bottom-up' approaches involving participation are more likely to achieve ownership and self-direction. This latter approach in relation to quality has been pioneered in the UK by Alison Kitson and Helen Kendall (1986) under the auspices of the Rcn's 'Standards of Care Project' which during the 1980s has been highly successful in empowering nurses to act, particularly in the area of setting standards.

Standard setting and criteria

The terms 'standard' and 'criteria' have already been used within this chapter and their relationship to values demonstrated, but how are they defined and what comes first?

Depending on the situation, the value or the problem may be the starting point. For example sometimes the exact standard is agreed verbally by everyone; it may just need writing down in terms of what is acceptable as a minimum level of performance. For example nurses working within a particular elderly care setting may feel strongly that the absolute minimum frequency that immobile patients in bed with sacral pressure sores should be turned is 2-hourly. This therefore reflects the minimum standard expected to be met when caring for patients in this client group. This does not mean however that it would be inappropriate to turn individual clients more frequently if judged necessary, and this would be prescribed on individual careplans.

At other times when looking at a particular problem it may be difficult to identify immediately what the standards are, and so one would first consider which criteria may be used to indicate the quality of a particular service. For example when considering the quality of the service provided by Health Visitors one could ask the question, what would indicate the quality of the service provided? One possible answer could include 'the uptake of children's immunizations'. Immunization uptake could therefore be one indicator or criterion by which the quality of the service given by health visitors could be considered. However if a standard was then combined with this criterion, then the following outcome standard could result:

> At least 95% of all children under the age of 5 within a particular locality have been immunised against whooping cough.

A criterion is therefore 'a value-free indicator' and Bloch (1977) defines it more formally as 'the value free name of a variable believed or known to be a relevant indicator of the quality of patient care,' and subsequently defines a standard as 'a desired and achievable level of performance corresponding with a criterion, against which actual performance can be judged'. The standard then is the 'yardstick' for comparison. This yardstick needs to be both explicit and consistent, just as when comparing venous pressure readings the yardstick for referencing the position of the right atrium could be either the sternal angle, or the fourth intercostal space mid-axilla. For the readings to be of any significance when compared, the same reference point must be consistently used. If explicit standards do not already exist then the starting point may be first to brainstorm the criteria thought to be relevant indicators of quality in a particular area, followed by the setting of agreed standards. Table 7.10 provides an illustration of this technique in relation to the question 'How would one know that individualised care was being given to patients in a ward where elderly people were being cared for?'

Table 7.10   Possible criteria which may be identified in response to the question, 'How do I know that individualised care is being given?' Examples of possible standards in relation to these criteria are also illustrated. (Manley 1991b)

Possible criteria	Standards
Careplans	Each careplan contains a reference as to how the patient likes to be addressed.
	Each careplan contains a statement in the patients own words of their expectations of care.
Organisational approach	Each patient can identify their own nurse.
Patients' activities of living	Each patient has different routines of daily living.
	Each patient has breakfast at a time negotiated with them.

Standards themselves therefore allow for nursing care to be judged from the point of view of whether the standard has been met or not; but a further essential element relates to *how* they are set. Several writers address this point, one being Crow (1981) who defines a standard of care as 'some measure or measures by which nursing care can be judged or compared, and where the measures used are agreed upon by common consent'. The first World Health Organization (WHO) meeting on the development of standards of nursing practice (cited Royal College of Nursing, 1984), and endorsed by the RCN also define a standard as an 'agreed upon level of care required for a particular purpose'.

The point that standards are 'agreed upon' and involve 'common consent' suggests that standards should be set in a participatory and consultatory way rather than as a 'top-down' process involving staff complying with the wishes of others. However, although there will always be some need for mandatory standards which are in fact policies, e.g., in relation to fire, health and safety, and infection control, these are usually relatively few in number.

For standards to be owned therefore they will need to be derived in a democratic and participatory way, and will represent areas of common ground in terms of individual personal values. But for standards to be of any relevance to practice they too need to fulfill certain criteria as identified by the WHO (cited Royal College of Nursing, 1984). They need to be:

reasonable
understandable
useful
measurable
observable
achievable.

Wilson (1987) too identifies similar criteria using the terms:

relevant
understandable
measurable
behavioural
achievable

Standards therefore need to be measurable and observable either directly or indirectly to facilitate their auditing. Wilson also recognises the need to involve staff in writing standards but emphasises the need to adapt policies and protocols rather than starting from scratch each time. Other aspects to consider when setting standards relate to whether they should be minimum, optimum or maximum in nature

(WHO cited Royal College of Nursing, 1984). The answer to this question would depend on the nature of the standard, the resources, and how it was to be audited. For example a standard relating to patient safety would be expected to be met in every single situation. It would therefore be a minimum standard and total compliance would always be expected. However a standard concerning patients' knowledge and understanding may not always be possible to achieve in every situation because of factors such as language difficulties, mental impairment, drugs and other influences. This may therefore represent a maximal standard, one that is being striven for in every situation but because of the exceptions mentioned, compliance to the standard would be expected to be less than 100 per cent if it was audited. A framework for setting standards at local level and their subsequent incorporation into a district index is outlined by Kitson and Kendall (1986) and illustrated in Fig. 7.2.

The actual writing of standards is further developed by the DySSSy approach (Royal College of Nursing, 1990) mentioned earlier. The actual steps involved in formulating standards using DySSSy include:

1.   Choosing a topic.
2.   Identifying a sub-topic.
3.   Defining the relevant care group.
4.   Formulating structure, process and outcome criteria.
5.   Obtaining management support.
6.   Setting implementation and review dates.

This approach also promotes and emphasises the fundamental value of ownership of standards by practitioners. Other principles underlying the DySSSy approach are outlined in Table 7.11.

Integral to the DySSSy method is the need for nurse management to be involved in some system of co-ordinating and indexing standards, as well as supporting the validity and realism of the standards set.

Table 7.11   Principles of the Dynamic Standard Setting System (DySSSy) (RCN 1990)

1. Owned and controlled by practitioners

2. Participation and involvement of practitioners

3. Patient/client focused

4. Situation-based

5. Sets achievable standards

6. Potentially multi-disciplinary

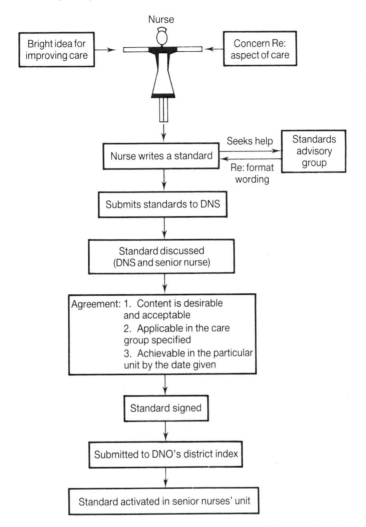

Fig. 7.2   The steps in developing local standards (Kitson, A. and
Kendall, H. (1986). Rest Assured. *Nursing Times*, August 27,
28–31).

Provision of support and facilitation from both management and
education are essential prerequisites if the whole nursing service is to
improve and maintain its quality. Setting standards in the absence of
careful and experienced support and facilitation can result in de-
moralised staff who after setting out with great enthusiasm wain
because their aspirations are not met, particularly if such aspirations
were too ambitious in the first instance. One method of ensuring that

staff's own identified goals can be met, is to proceed in small incremental steps as proposed by Lindblom (1959). Lindblom describes how people actually make successful decisions, rather than prescribing how they should make decisions in an ideal world. Such an approach can still enable rapid change, as each small incremental step can be passed through quickly. This is because the objectives at each stage are easily achievable, subsequently demoralisation is not so likely to occur.

On these lines the approach used by the author is outlined in Table 7.12. The topic area is always selected by the staff who agree to write the standards, this would vary according to the areas of concern identified by staff, and their personal interest and/or expertise. The

---

Table 7.12 Incremental goal orientated steps in the standard setting process. (Manley 1991c)

Stage 1	Identify topic area of interest with the facilitator.
Stage 2	Collect resources about the topic including use of the literature, using various experts, and other resources already available.
Stage 3	Meet with the facilitator and collectively write draft outcome standards, performance standards and identify specific resources for a particular client group.
Stage 4	Identify in depth rationales and key references to support performance and structural standards. These can then contribute to education and management in terms of individual performance review (IPR) and through making the knowledge for action explicit.
Stage 5	Type draft standards using a wordprocessor. This facilitates change following consultation, and also later updating.
Stage 6	Circulate standards to all members of the unit/ward nursing team for comment.
Stage 7	If outcome standards reflect contributions from other professionals then ownership may be obtained by openly discussing them with the respective groups or preferably involving them in the process from the beginning.
Stage 8	Complete the final draft following agreement by all involved. Identify how the standards can be included into orientation, job and performance review processes.
Stage 9	Consider how and who will audit outcome standards, and how frequently they need to be audited.

time interval for each step is negotiated, thus recognising individual and organisational constraints on time. Outcome standards are identified first as these are of paramount importance to the client, and it is these which will later be audited. But it is the process (or performance standards) which are essential to identify in terms of clarifying staff roles and performance expectations, rationales for action, as well as providing the basis of learning outcomes and competencies for students.

Outcome standards involving other disciplines also need to be owned by these disciplines from the beginning. Such ownership can be achieved by formulating multi-disciplinary statements of values and beliefs from which standards can then be derived, or by using multi-disciplinary group problem-solving techniques such as Quality Circles.

Outcomes

As far as clients and patients are concerned, the outcomes of the service that we seek to provide are probably the most important part. It is the achievement of positive outcomes which is the reason that clients use the service. Marek (1989) defines outcome from a nursing perspective as 'a measurable change in a client's health status related to the receipt of nursing care'. This definition however implies that it is easy to separate out nursing's contribution to changes in health status from the contribution made by other professions, which is in fact very difficult to do. Hamric (1989) considers that 'it is difficult to identify outcome criteria solely attributable to nursing care', and that the areas in which nursing may be able to make a unique contribution are those concerning cognitive, behavioural and psychosocial variables, although these are more difficult to measure than health status. This link may be easier to establish when nursing is the sole contributor to health care, as can be found in organisations possessing nursing beds. But in most situations, nurses function as one of a team of professions involved in health care. This multi-disciplinary approach to care is the essence of post-Griffiths management (Strong and Robinson, 1988) where the emphasis is on the total service rendered to the client, rather than the fragmented part played by single professions.

The work of Brooten *et. al.* (1986) studied the outcome of early hospital discharge on low birth weight infants whose families received clinical nurse specialist support, demonstrating it to be both safe and cost-effective. This study illustrates a link between the activities (process) of the clinical nurse specialist and outcome, but it also links collaborative multi-disciplinary team-work to outcome. This relationship between good collaborative teamwork and positive patient outcome is also demonstrated in other studies (Knaus *et. al.*, 1986).

Outcomes are therefore currently very much in vogue in terms of general management. This is because they enable judgements to be made about the effectiveness and appropriateness of the health care services being provided. Of course this involves the combined efforts of all the professions involved in the provision of health care, not just one. Consider the elderly person who improves and becomes self-caring again following hospital admission for a chest infection with associated hypoxia-induced disorientation and confusion; how was this positive outcome achieved, and which profession is responsible? A whole range of interventions or influencing factors may have accounted for the improvement, e.g.:

(a)   the antibiotics prescribed by the doctor.
(b)   the trusting relationship developed by the nurse which enabled successful communication, teaching, understanding, and compliance in taking medications.
(c)   the chest physiotherapy administered by the physiotherapists.
(d)   the supportive family, participating in care.
(e)   the patient's positive attitude of mind.
(f)   the catering staff's well presented and nutritionally balanced food.

Hence one can see how difficult it is to identify how the outcome is influenced by the actions of any single provider, let alone any one profession involved in care delivery (Spross, 1989). However, focussing on outcomes could be considered a positive advantage if it means that professions have to communicate with each other and agree on the outcomes being strived for as a team, rather than as different professions. Once agreement is achieved then common aims and objectives can result in improved performance and increased understanding of each others role. Common agreement is more difficult at Health Authority level but at unit/ward level is much easier to achieve because patients with similar needs tend to be cared for together. Such common aims are achieved by first identifying common values, beliefs and purposes.

Another benefit of focussing on outcomes is that it forces one to address exactly what is trying to be achieved, therefore clarifying purpose rather than just focussing on actions. For example a ward manager may be concerned about the lack of cleanliness of the floors, and this may be an overriding priority problem to address. However, if standard setting commences with outcomes then it would be the purpose of having clean floors that is emphasised. For example the purpose may be to minimise the nosocomial urinary catheter infection rate (because urinary catheter bags are near the floor), or the number of accidents occurring due to wet or cluttered floors. In this example then it would be the outcome criteria of urinary catheter infection rates, and accident rates that would act as the starting point in identifying outcome standards.

Hence one of the difficulties in developing outcome indicators is that they are affected by such a multitude of factors, often not controllable. Secondly, it is very difficult to demonstrate the relationship of actions to outcome. Most of us suspect that clinical areas with excellent reputations for high standards of care have good outcomes but this relationship is not too easy to actually demonstrate. Audrey Miller's (1985) work demonstrated such a relationship in care of the elderly wards that used the nursing process where patients were in hospital for more than a month. The outcome criterion involved was the patient dependency level, which she demonstrated was reduced in the clinical areas using the nursing process with patients resident for longer than one month.

The third difficulty is the development of outcome indicators that reflect accurately the quality of care, that is, indicators which are valid. This is complicated by the problem that quality of care is difficult to measure because it is such a broad concept which as previously indicated is also difficult to define. It can be easier to use indicators that are quantifiable, e.g., discharge rates. But do such indicators reflect quality of care? Contradictions are well recognised; e.g., discharge rates are not considered in conjunction with re-admission rates. Throughput or bed occupancy are other examples of easily quantifiable indicators which may reflect the efficiency of the service rather than its effectiveness. Such rates do not indicate whether it is the same patient who has been re-admitted six times, or six different patients admitted once, the latter scenario being more indicative of a quality service than the first. Efficiency and effectiveness are therefore concepts which relate to the quantitive and qualititive indicators commonly used.

Defining and classifying outcomes

Rinke (1988, cited by Marek, 1989) identifies five key dimensions of outcome which have been further analysed by Marek. These are explained in Table 7.13.

Wilson (1987) considers the nature of outcome encompasses the three elements of quantity, quality and client satisfaction. In the latter it is well recognised that although perceptions of clients may be good, when compared with professional standards of practice there may be a discrepancy (Wilson, 1987). Hamric (1989) also advises caution when using patient satisfaction as an indicator of nursing care quality. This is because in the United States it is a potent area for competition, where hospitals are competing against each other for patients, through

Table 7.13 Key aspects of outcome and synonymous concepts as identified by Rinke (1988, cited Marek 1989)

Key aspect	Synonymn	Explanation
1. Change	Result Consequence Effect Product	A difference, alteration, improvement in a client or client response as a result of intervention.
2. Client	Individual Family Targeted Group Community	The recipient of the service and focus of outcome measurement.
3. Health	Wellbeing	Health is the phenomena in which change is to occur and may include aspects of physical, psychological, behavioural, spiritual and functional well-being.
4. Relation		This assumes a relationship between nursing intervention and outcome.
5. Health Care Service		The health care service is the process which effects change, or causes an outcome.

marketing 'consumer comfort and accessibility'. Specifically, Hamric cites Eriksen's (1987) study which demonstrated a predominantly inverse relationship between the quality of nursing care and patient satisfaction, particularly in the areas of physical care and teaching patients to deal with their illnesses. The reason suggested by Eriksen (1987) for this was that professional nursing values are at times in opposition to those of the patients.

Outcomes referred to in the past have usually focused on negative attributes such as those identified by Lohr (1988) who labelled them the five 'D's; death, disease, disability, discomfort and dissatisfaction, rather than benefits such as satisfaction, quality of life, independence and survival rates. Outcomes may also differ in scope, their focus being specific, broad or generic (Marek, 1989). Examples which demonstrate this scope are illustrated in Table 7.14.

Table 7.14 Scope of outcome and examples (after Marek 1989)

Scope	Focus	Example
Specific	Relate to a particular nursing/ medical diagnosis or problem.	Resolution of specific nursing diagnosis.
Broad	Apply to a large category of clients.	Accessibility of community patients to district nurses at weekends.
Generic	Apply to all clients of health care system.	Mortality and morbidity rates Safety Rehospitalisation

A further aspect important to recognise is the time interval at which outcomes are evaluated (Wright, 1984; Marek, 1989), as 'there is relatively little knowledge of the best time to measure an outcome indicator' (Marek, 1989). In relation to health status for example some changes may only be temporary, but others may have longer duration, while patients too may also have different rates of recovery (Waters, 1986). Outcome indicators used to measure the quality of nursing care have been crudely classified into groups by Marek (1989) as indicated in Table 7.15.

Process standards

'People may want to do well but are limited by the structures, systems and resources within which they work', or in many cases 'by their lack of knowledge of what constitutes good quality, and the lack of any means of knowing whether they are achieving it'. (Morris, 1989). Certainly, knowing what is expected and also how to do what is expected, is the first stage in converting knowledge into competent action. Competence itself has been linked to quality of care by Shukla (1981) in a replication study comparing team nursing with primary nursing. Shukla first raised the level of competency in both control and experimental groups by providing an educational input. Once a high level of competency had been achieved in both groups as measured by the Slater Nursing Competency Rating Scale (Wandelt and Stewart, 1975), then primary nursing was introduced into the experimental group. Shukla demonstrated that the quality of care using the Quality Patient Care Scale (Qualpacs) (Wandelt and Ager, 1974) increased in both groups, and that this was attributed predominantly to increasing the competency of staff, rather than through practising primary nursing, although some effect was also attributed to primary nursing.

Table 7.15 Types of outcome indicators used to measure the quality of care in nursing (after Marek 1989)

Types of outcome criteria	Specific outcome criterion
Psychosocial Client's patterns of behaviour, communication, and relationships.	coping attitudes behaviour communication social interaction application of skills motivation
Quality of life Or 'well-being'	health* comfort* stereotyped behaviour* proximal experience* relationships* focus* developmental appropriateness of environment* sense of personal worth*
Physiological status Processes which maintain life	skin integrity vital signs weight wound healing
Functional Activities of daily living, mobility and communication	activities of daily living mobility self-care
Behaviour domain Activities, skills and actions of clients	knowledge skills compliance motivation
Symptom control	pain comfort fatigue nausea constipation
Patient satisfaction	'focus' more on the art of care rather than the technical aspects' (Marek 1989)
Home maintenance Functioning of family in the home environment of the client.	family living patterns environment support roles

Table 7.15 – *Continued*

Types of outcome criteria	Specific outcome criterion
Goal attainment	attainment of expected outcomes
Safety	maintenance of safety
Nursing diagnosis	resolution of nursing diagnosis – is identified by Marek as potentially a powerful tool in evaluating nursing outcome.

* Specific outcome indicators identified by Robinson (1987) for people with a mental handicap.

To answer Donabedian's (1966) question 'is good nursing care being carried out?' one has to first identify what good nursing is. This involves identifying explicitly the actions and knowledge expected of nurses in specific areas of practice. It is process (performance) standards that fulfill this purpose. Process standards encompass the following aspects:

1. Knowledge, attitudes, values and beliefs possessed.
2. Assessment actions.
3. Planning actions.
4. Implementation of care.
5. Evaluation of care.

The broad minimum standards expected of registered nurses are outlined in the competencies required for registration with the UKCC. But it is the value and beliefs held about the nature of nursing which will specifically influence the type of knowledge and skills deemed appropriate. These values and beliefs also provide direction about what nurses assess, and their role in intervention. (*see* Chapter 4) Different conceptual models in nursing encapsulate specific values and beliefs about the role and purpose of nursing; the nature of the environment or society; the nature of the individual person and the nature of health (*see* Chapter 5). Each nursing model will focus on and emphasise different aspects. Conceptual models therefore suggest even more specifically the actions and knowledge expected of nurses (Manley, 1991a). These expectations however would be derived from the nursing team's own philosophy, through choosing a conceptual model (or parts of a model) which are congruent with it.

Buswell (1986 cited Keighley, 1989) considers that the actual process of care delivery can be viewed from two perspectives, **technical performance** and **expressive performance**. The technical aspect of performance can be 'both measured and controlled corporately' (Keighley, 1989) and encompasses:

1. The effectiveness with which operational aspects are performed.
2. The knowledge of procedures.
3. The effective and efficient utilisation of technology and equipment.

Expressive performance in contrast 'is concerned with the attitudes of staff, with their relationships and interactions . . . and with the manner in which the staff delivers the service' (Keighley, 1989). This is much more difficult to measure, but Keighley suggests that expressive performance is more influential than technical performance in terms of consumer perceptions of quality. So if expressive performance is poor even if technical performance is good, then the consumer will consider poor quality care has been received. A more serious scenario however would be one where the consumer perceives the quality of care to be high because expressive performance is high, even though technical performance is low. Technical and expressive performance are both important components of nursing. Technical performance can be specified through performance standards, but it is through Individual Performance Review (IPR), and the subsequent access to educational resources for personal development that both technical and expressive performance can be developed in individual staff members. Systems for IPR are therefore essential prerequisites if both technical and expressive performance standards are to be improved within any organisation.

Structural standards

Structural standards specify the quantity and quality of the inputs into the health care system. Specifically Donabedian (1980) would identify these as the people, equipment and the environment. The World Health Organisation (cited by Healy, 1988) too, include these components in their definition of structure:

> 'the characteristics of the providers of care, of the tools and resources at their disposal, and of the physical and organisational settings in which they work.'

The organisational environment itself is under the control of management. Smith-Marker (1988) considers that structural standards provide the foundation of any organisation through policy, and that management is responsible for formulating and shaping that policy.
Table 7.16 illustrates criteria and examples of existing standards or

Table 7.16 Criteria and possible examples of standards derived from Donabedian's (1980) three components of structure

Structural component	Criteria	Examples of areas for development/ existence of standards
People	Number of nursing staff	Various patient and client dependency classification systems determine optimum staffing establishments in relation to patient dependency, e.g., the Telford System (1979), the Cheltenham Method (Cheltenham and District Health Authority 1982), and Criteria for Care (Ball, Goldstone and Collier, 1984)
	Skill mix	Stated number of establishment posts at each grade for each clinical area
	Specialists	The provision of for example, infection control nurses, stomatherapists, bereavement counsellors, aromatherapists, staff counsellors, nurse practitioners (*see* Chapter 3)
Equipment	Health and safety policies	No smoking policies in the proximity of oxygen supplies. Policies regarding the provision of hoists for lifting patients, and the provision of 'sharps' boxes and handwashing facilities
	Equipment function	For example, policies regarding resuscitation equipment and electrical equipment
	Number/type of equipment	For example, the number of electrical thermometers, the range of oxygen humidifiers available, or specialised pressure-reducing beds
Environment	Health and safety policies	Temperature of the environment. Provision of patient privacy. Infection control policies
	Educational resources	The provision of orientation, developmental and updating programmes

Table 7.16 – *Continued*

Structural component	Criteria	Examples of areas for development/ existence of standards
	Information systems	The provision of information for example about infection rates, outcomes, staff retention, patient/ client satisfaction, screening, and local population profile (*see* Chapter 6)
	Systems for IPR	The organisational environment and the necessary educational and documentation facilities to support IPR

areas for development, derived from the three components of structure identified by Donabedian (1980).

Monitoring and measuring

Monitoring, evaluation and audit are terms that are important to
understand in the context of this section. The World Health Organization (cited by Healy, 1988) considers **evaluation** to be:

> 'the systematic and scientific process of determining the extent to
> which a planned intervention or programme achieves predeter-
> mined goals.'

this is different from **monitoring**, which is defined as:

> 'the ongoing measurements of a variety of health care indicators of
> quality to identify potential problems.'
>   (World Health Organization cited by Healy, 1988)

Evaluation and monitoring therefore differ in terms of **when** they
occur. The difference is explained by Dickens (1990) who suggests that
evaluation relates to a single point in time, and monitoring is ongoing.
Bergman (1982) in her definition of evaluation emphasises **what**
evaluation of care is, defining it as:

> 'objective measurement of concrete phenomena, as well as sub-
> jective perceptions and opinions of the "feeling" of nursing care as
> reported by recipients, providers, and important others.'

This definition therefore supports the need for collecting both quantitative and qualitative data, and the involvement of all who participate in the giving and receiving of care. (*see* Chapter 1 for greater insight into the nature of care).

Audit as a word has its origins in accountancy and simply means the verification and examination of accounts. This task involves a formal check that accounts are correct. The origin of its use in health care is reflected in the World Health Organization's (cited by Healy, 1988) definition. This describes medical audit, stating it to be the 'retrospective examination of the clinical application of medical knowledge as revealed by the medical record.' Within nursing also, the word audit has been related to the documentation of care, for example the Phaneuf Nursing Audit (1964) involved the analysis of nursing records and the findings were correlated with quality of care. The Australian Council on Hospital Standards (cited by Healy, 1988) in their definition of medical audit however use the term much more broadly and encompass different methods of evaluation of quality, therefore implying that audit does not just apply to documentation. The same group however, when defining nursing audit again focus only on records defining it as 'the systematic review of records in order to evaluate the quality of nursing care . . . ' The use of the word 'audit' in terms of the documentation of care therefore relates to the verification and examination of care that has already been given, through the examination of documentation. This is called **retrospective audit**, which also encompasses other methods besides the examination of records, such as observation techniques. **Concurrent audit** in contrast is the term associated with the verification and examination of care at the time it actually is given, and it too involves the use of tools which may utilise a range of methods. However, regardless of whether audit is performed retrospectively or concurrently certain assumptions are common to both and these are:

1. That actual standards of performance already exist.
2. That these standards have been agreed.
3. These standards are explicit, and
4. They are in a form that can be easily verified.

So to summarise, the simple purpose of audit is the verification of standards in a specifically defined area to establish whether they are being met or not. Whether care is audited retrospectively or concurrently, whether care is monitored or evaluated, the range of methods available for fulfilling these functions can be classified into the following groups:

1. Auditing documentation.
2. Direct observation.

3.   Interviews and/or questionnaires.
4.   Combinations of the above.

These methods are formal approaches to evaluating, monitoring and auditing care. However, less formal approaches which emphasise individual development and performance are becoming increasingly more common and important to the development of professional nursing practice. Such methods include individual reflection on practice, and peer review.

Approaches to evaluating, monitoring and auditing individual performance

The reflective practitioner

'The Reflective Practitioner' is a phrase coined by Donald Schön (1983), an American professor of urban studies and education. This phrase epitomises the professional qualities expected of British nurses in forthcoming decades and as reflected in Project 2000 curricula. Schön's work recognises the importance of knowledge based in practice and reflection-in-action, and how these approaches can help individuals to try out solutions in their practice and use the knowledge gained to contribute to future practice. Thinking and doing cannot be separated (Schön, 1983), and so through repeated and continuous reflection and evaluation of personal practice, individual performance continues to develop and grow.

Peer review

Peer review is a tool by which individual nurses can evaluate their practice. 'A peer is a colleague of equal rank' (Ciske, Verhey and Egan, 1983). However Leibold (1983) defines more fully its meaning when referring to clinical nurse specialists review as:

> 'the critical evaluation of one's clinical practice by colleagues who are equal in education, qualifications and/or position and therefore are able to make qualitative judgements concerning clinical performance.'

Such an approach therefore permits the evaluation and improvement of performance and facilitates individual accountability to the consumer of the service. As an approach it is central to the practice of primary nursing as well as quality assurance and the maintenance of performance standards. Peer Review was first promoted as a means of maintaining standards in nursing in 1972 by the American Nurses' Association in response to the recognition that nurses needed to be accountable for, and responsible to the public for their practice. Peer review according to Winch (1989) stems from the medical literature of the 1960s. He considers that peer review, to be successful, must be built on and evolve from peer support which exists when there are opportunities for constructive feedback related to role performance and encouragement of professional growth.

Wilson (1987) considers that peer review is preferable to other types of evaluation particularly 'top-down' methods, for the following three reasons:

1. Reviews by practitioners of practitioners are more likely to be accurate than evaluation performed by people who no longer practice that which is under review.
2. There is an opportunity for practitioners to reinforce their own standards when evaluating the practice of colleagues.
3. It demonstrates that 'quality belongs to the practitioners, and not to management.'

The role of management is therefore a facilitative one, and one that creates an environment in which peer review is fostered and nurtured. Ramphal (1974) identified two types of peer review, that involving the evaluation of the quality of care given by an individual, and secondly, that given by an agency, for example a specific nursing team.

Winch (1989) recognises two major factors which influence the success of peer review. One is the establishment of trust, the other is the reduction of professional passivity. Winch considers there to be the risk of negative punitive connotations with peer review which can make it unsuccessful. However, through the establishment of trust which Winch identifies is akin to peer support, and through emphasising the fact that 'peer review evaluates job-specific performance criteria and not personal characteristics or worth' this danger can be overcome. The second factor, professional passivity, is also related to the first factor and can be recognised as reluctance and unwillingness to pass judgement on another. Peer review practices can be initiated through presentations of patients' nursing care. This is integral to the practice of primary nursing where colleagues of the primary nurse are encouraged to constructively challenge and discuss selected interventions, as well as providing additional ideas in the management of specific problems that patients may have.

Individual performance review

Individual performance review (IPR) is a two-way process involving post-holders and their managers. This approach involves sharing and clarifying job expectations and purpose, mutually identifying needs and negotiating personal action plans in relation to both the personal development and performance of the post holder. This plan is then reviewed usually yearly but sometimes more frequently, and if necessary modified. Performance standards may be incorporated into this process as they specifically identify expected performance in specific areas of practice. Orientation periods for new post-holders provide ideal opportunities for introducing employees to this process. Action plans would be unique to the individual post-holder as each person commencing a new job would have their own repertoire of skills and knowledge, and also different backgrounds in terms of experience and practice. Each individual would therefore have a unique personal profile and differing areas for development. The National Health Service Training Authority (1987) identify three stages in the IPR cycle:

1. Job clarification.
2. Monitoring.
3. Major Performance Review.

Each stage is related to the other through the personal action/ development plan, which can be revised if necessary by negotiation if job expectations change and different skills and knowledge are subsequently required. IPR therefore provides an invaluable opportunity for personal reflection, monitoring and auditing in mutual conjunction with managers. Managers therefore besides facilitating this process also have responsibility for providing the necessary resources and educational opportunities to allow the individual post-holder to develop.

The Slater Nursing Competencies Rating Scale

The Slater Nursing Competencies Rating Scale (Wandelt and Stewart, 1975) is a tool which can be used to provide information about individual performance, specifically the quality of care delivered by individual nurses to patients and clients. A total of 84 items are included in the scale which are grouped into the following six sections:

Psycho-social: Individual.
Psycho-social: Group.
Physical.

General.
Communication.
Professional implications.

Individuals are observed by trained raters who make judgements about interactions observed between patients and individual nurses, or on behalf of clients. Observed performance is then mentally compared with the performance expected of a first level nurse and a score of 1–5 attributed. This tool can be used either on the spot or retrospectively over a period of time. It has been demonstrated to be valid and reliable in general medical, surgical, paedaetric and psychiatric settings if at least 60 of the 84 items have been observed in a minimum period of two hours observation. Generally as a tool it has been used predominantly in a more formal way, or to research different approaches to care and or educational preparation. It does lend itself for use between peers but would require a time investment in learning how to use the tool.

Shukla's study (1981) mentioned earlier suggests the major influence that personal competency has on the quality of care. It therefore further supports the strategy of investing in individual development as a method of maintaining and improving quality of care provided to clients. The mechanism involved may be the improvement of both technical and expressive performance. The items in the rating scale itself represent collections of performance standards.

Approaches to evaluating, monitoring and auditing performance of the nursing service

Several tools were developed particularly in the 1970s in the United States to measure quality of care provided by specific nursing services at clinical level. Such tools are well known and include the following examples:

The Quality Patient Care Scale (QUALPACS) (Wandelt and Ager, 1974).
The Phaneuf Audit (Phaneuf, 1964).
The Rush-medicus Index (Hegyvary and Haussmann, 1976).
Monitor (in the UK) (Goldstone, Ball and Collier, 1984).

Several other tools exist and these are comprehensively outlined in the Bibliography of Nursing Quality Assurance and Standards of Care: 1932–87 collated and annotated by Kitson and Harvey (1991). This text is particularly recommended to the reader as an essential reference handbook regarding the history and development of quality assurance in nursing.

The tools outlined above predominantly focus on quality indicators concerning the process of care and/or its documentation, although Monitor does also address aspects of structure and outcome. Other important tools include measures of outcome such as patient satisfaction and health care status as discussed earlier in the section on outcome standards.

One last important area to include in this section is the auditing of standards through the measurement of compliance. Some standards can be measured directly because they lend themselves to yes or no answers to the question, Is the standard being met? Other standards may not be quite so simple to audit and therefore require the design of audit tools which determine whether a particular standard is being met or not. An additional aspect to consider in the process of measuring standards is whether the standard is of a minimum, optimal, or maximal nature as this would have a bearing on the level of compliance expected. In other words, if the standard is expected to be met on every occasion, then 100 per cent compliance would be expected. On the other hand, if the standard is of a maximal nature, then a lower compliance may be acceptable. Alternatively, there may be a need to gradually improve a particular standard as a more realistic way to achieve it. In this instance the compliance rating may be increased over a period of time to reflect this progression. Once standards have been set and agreed, aspects such as compliance factors and auditing need to be carefully considered. However many of the problems of auditing standards can be reduced or avoided if thoughts about how the standard can be audited are kept in mind during their initial design.

Identifying choices and action planning

Quality circles

Lees and Dale (1989) state that 'action is a process not a single step'. One way of addressing situations that require action is through involving all staff in the quest for improving quality. In situations where there are problems with maintaining standards and subsequently poor staff morale, 'Quality Circles' may be a useful strategy to consider. Quality Circles as a technique has been increasingly used within health care settings in the UK. Its use is well researched by Lees and Dale of the Manchester School of Management (1989). This trend is reflected by the establishment of the National Society of Quality Circles in 1982 and the subsequent production of a training manual by the King's Fund to guide leaders and facilitators in 1986 (King's Fund, 1986). Quality Circles however depend on the willingness of representatives from all disciplines involved in a particular area of care to participate in such a process. As a method it allows active participation in both the identification of solutions to problems and their subsequent implementation, thus fostering 'a personal commitment to the quality' of the service (Newcomb and Kleiner, 1989). Quality Circles can be defined as:

> 'a process whereby staff at every layer in an organisation work together as a team to improve quality of service and work life.'
>
> (Hyde, 1984)

Stages in Quality Circles include:

1. Appointment of a facilitator – 'a person to be inside the circle but able to look objectively at the work and guide circle members through the traumas to come.'
2. Formation of a group of volunteers (5–10 is optimum) who meet once a week for an hour. A leader will emerge from the group.
3. First meeting – a brainstorming session to identify work related problems or areas for improved performance.
4. Analysis of problems thereby identifying which problems to deal with first.
5. Brainstorming possible solutions which are analysed.
6. Action by circle if authorised.
7. Presentation to management.

(Hyde, 1984)

Quality Circles constitute a problem-solving process which has a six-stage plan:

1. The problem.
2. Thorough investigation of the causes of the problem.
3. The solution.
4. The benefits to patients and staff.
5. Implementation.
6. Evaluation.

(Robson, 1988)

In Lees and Dale's study of the use of Quality Circles in a health authority based in the Midlands, the type of problems identified tended to fall into two groups, either they were:

(a) 'everyday management problems which tended to have more than one solution'.
(b) 'a huge problem which needed breaking down into manageable parts'.

Benefits identified by Lees and Dale in their study included improved patient care, noticeable improvements in staff morale, and greater teamwork. Training in Quality Circles techniques is essential if maximum benefit is to be obtained.

A unit based quality assurance model: the marker model

The Marker model (Smith-Marker, 1988) of quality assurance is a model which can be used at any level of health care be that at operational, unit or district level. It is a system that recognises there are many practices and aspects to quality assurance, and tries to bring these together in a co-ordinated and consistent way to produce a portfolio of all quality assurance activities in one place within a manual. This approach uses Donabedian's framework of structure, process and outcome, and is also dependent on the participative approaches encouraged by both DySSSy (Royal College of Nursing, 1990) and Wilson (1987), and although it may require modification for use in the UK its main attributes are that it was designed primarily for clinical practice settings. Secondly, it provides a consistent and explicit framework for co-ordinating standards. Structure, process and outcome standards are seen by Smith-Marker to be placed in a hierarchy as represented below in Fig. 7.3.

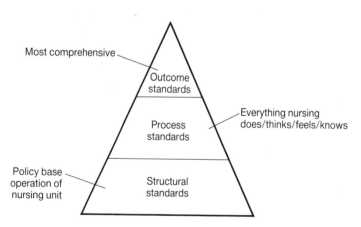

Fig. 7.3 Structural, process and outcome standards as a hierarchy. (Smith-Marker, 1988)

Structural standards define a) how the nursing system operates, and b) policy at all levels, whereas process standards have the following characteristics:

1. Defines actions, knowledge, skills of staff giving care.
2. Defines what constitutes care.
3. Are directed at the patient or the nurse.

Structure and process standards have explicit components in the Marker Model and these are identified in Tables 7.17 and 7.18.

The writing style and other suggestions about how these structural standards should be written are stipulated by Smith-Marker as:

1. Brief and succinct.
2. Thorough and covering all nine points.
3. Policies are outlined from the broad to the specific.
4. Each has an identified date for when they are written, and also a method of review.
5. Must be consistent with existing policies within the system.

The difference particularly between the last four formats of process standards within the Marker Model can be demonstrated by the following example concerning catheterisation of the bladder; a procedure would focus on the psychomotor steps involved in introducing a urinary catheter into the bladder, and would be directed at the nurse. A protocol would specify how a patient/client with a urinary catheter would be cared for in relation to this device, and so focuses on the patient. Guidelines would specify how and what would be documented in relation to fluid input and output. Standards of care may look at the needs of a specific client group, for example those who may be intermittently catheterising themselves. All would include performance standards.

   Outcome is seen by Smith-Marker (1988) to be applied to the four situations of

1. Staff development.
2. Patient education.
3. Quality assurance.
4. Care planning.

This area is probably the one requiring greater development within the model.

Total quality management

Total quality management is the 'philosophy of getting things right first time throughout the organisation, not just concentrating on the end product or service' (Morris, 1989), and is based on the assumption that

Table 7.17   The nine elements of structural standards identified at unit level. (Smith-Marker 1988)

Element	Components of element
Description of unit	a) Location, size, number of beds b) Patient population/acuity c) Type of unit e.g. rehabilitative, acute.
Purpose of unit	Purpose and philosophy
Overall objectives of unit	These are derived from the philosophy and would include: a) nursing-medical management e.g. a 'collaborative multi-disciplinary approach' b) environment c) equipment e.g. the equipment required to control pain or promote comfort. d) data collection e.g. patients length of stay, bed occupancy rate etc. e) research/teaching objectives
Administration/organis-ational approach	a) Organisational chart and narrative b) Policy statements (i) Nursing direction (ii) Medical direction (iii) Committee structure e.g. liaison/interprofessional and representatives.
Hours of operation	a) Normal b) Emergency
Criteria for admission and discharge	Relates to when and how patients are admitted, who can admit patients and what happens when demand for beds outstrips supply, and other issues concerned with admission.
Governing policies	a) general safety e.g. visitors, noise accidents b) electrical safety and maintenance c) infection control d) patient valuables e) confidentiality and patients rights f) emergency equipment and supplies g) patient support services e.g. laboratories, diagnostic facilities h) fire and disaster plans

Table 7.17 – *Continued*

Element	Components of element

Staffing of unit	a) establishment
	b) skill mix
	c) organisational approach e.g. primary, team nursing
	d) preparation of staff
	    (i) selection
	    (ii) orientation
	    (iii) continuing education
	    (iv) performance, peer review, individual performance review

Nursing responsibilities	By staff groups e.g. primary nurse, associate nurse etc or by grade e.g. 'D' grade. 'F' grade.

'the creation of quality services requires organisational and attitude change on the part of the service staff, with a strong lead being given on the part of the managers of the service' (Dickens, 1990). This philosophy is different from that which has predominantly influenced industry and also now health care, where the focus is on finding out what has gone right or wrong after the event through using various reviews, surveys and audits. Morris goes on to identify that the prerequisites to successful total quality management are:

Table 7.18   The six formats of process standards (Smith-Marker, 1988)

Job descriptions	Provide an overview of what position entails.
Performance standards	Define specific expectations of behaviour, knowledge and skill.
Procedures	Relate to the stages involved in specific psychomotor skills.
Protocols	Define the nursing management of broad patient problems or issues.
Guidelines	Specify how information and data is documented.
Standards of care	Define care for groups of patients for whom generalisations and predictions can be made because they share common problems and needs.

1. Being able to identify what the purpose of the service is, the needs of the consumer of the service and the provider of the service at every level.
2. Having positive attitudes about the importance of producing a quality service by staff working within the service at every level.
3. Displaying positive and active management of quality which requires
   - commitment from senior management
   - effective leadership
   - effective teamwork and team building.
4. 'recognition that quality involves considerably more tasks and activities than the direct treatment of patients' (Morris, 1989).

Although nurses are at the interface between the patient and the service, this approach recognises that there are many sequences of activities further back down the chain that will influence the sort of service that nurses can give. An example that highlights this point well can be seen when there are problems with the supply and distribution of clean linen, particularly at weekends and bank holidays, resulting in scarcity of linen in clinical areas for the provision of patients. Total quality management recognises the importance of every link in the chain. This perspective has implications for nursing in two ways:

1. Attempts to maintain quality cannot be carried out in isolation from other disciplines.

Everyone involved in the process needs to participate in the process. For example, standards involving transfer of patients from a ward to the operating room must also include participation of the porters.

2. Working together in planning for quality has several benefits:
   (a) improved team work.
   (b) ownership of standards which will therefore be more likely to be implemented.
   (c) better understanding and more insight in to each others role and function.

Total Quality Management is therefore about obtaining total commitment to producing a quality service by everyone working in the organisation at all levels of function.

Conclusion

This chapter has tried to introduce the breadth of concern encompassed by quality assurance through attempting to integrate perspectives particularly from both the disciplines of nursing and management. It cannot claim to be totally comprehensive in its subject matter, but hopefully it has provided a framework and some superficial insight by which to understand quality issues and quality assurance.

It is hoped that this will stimulate the reader's interest in the subject and encourage the reader to progress further by reflecting on the personal contribution that they can make in the quest for excellence in nursing through firstly making explicit and acknowledging the characteristics of good practice within nursing; and secondly, by initiating and maintaining quality assurance practices as members of a collaborative health care team. The purpose of it all being the provision of a better service to our patients and clients.

References

American Nurses' Association. (1977). *Guidelines for Review of Nursing Care at the Local Level.* ANA, Kansas City.

American Nurses' Association and Sutherland Learning Associates. (1982). *Professional Nurses' Role in Quality Assurance.* ANA, Kansas City. (Nursing quality assurance management learning system vol. 1).

Ball, J. A., Goldstone, L. A. and Collier, M. M. (1984). *Criteria for Care: the Manual of the North West Staffing Levels Project.* Newcastle upon Tyne Polytechnic Products, Newcastle upon Tyne.

Baker, N. C., Cerone, S. B., Gaze, N. and Knapp, T. P. (1984). The effect of type of thermometer and length of time inserted on oral temperature measurements of afebrile subjects. *Nursing Research*, **33(2)** 109–11.

Bergman, R. (1982). Evaluation of nursing care – could it make a difference? *International Journal of Nursing Studies*, **19(2)**, 53–60.

Bloch, D. (1977). Criteria, standards, norms – crucial terms in quality assurance. *Journal of Nursing Administration*, **7(7)**, 20–30.

Bloch, D. (1980). Interrelated issues in evaluation and evaluation research; a researcher's perspective. *Nursing Research*, **29(2)**, 69–73.

Brenner, R. (1985). Setting standards. *Nursing Times*, **81(45)**, 26–8.

British Standards Institute. (1979). *Glossary of Terms Used in Quality Assurance.* BSI, Milton Keynes. (BS4778).

British Standards Institute. (1987). *Guide to Quality Management and Quality Systems Management.* BSI Milton Keynes.

Brooten, D., Kumar, S., Brown, L. P., Butts, P., Finkler, S. A., Bakewell-Sachs, S., Gibbons, A. and Delivoria-Papadopoulos, M. (1986). A randomised clinical trial of early hospital discharge and home follow-up of very low-birth-weight infants. *New England Journal of Medicine*. **315(15)**, 934–9.

Campbell, J., Finch, D., Allport, C., Erickson, H. and Swain, A. P. (1985). A theoretical approach to nursing assessment. *Journal of Advanced Nursing*, **10(2)**, 111–5.

Cheltenham and District Health Authority. (1982). *Report of the Working Party on Total Care Nursing Dependency Study at Cheltenham General Hospital*. Cheltenham and District HA, Cheltenham.

Ciske, K. L., Verhey, C. A. and Egan, E. C. (1983). Improving peer relationships through contracting in primary nursing. *Journal of Nursing Administration*, **13(2)**, 5–9.

Crow, R. A. (1981). Research and the standards of nursing care: what is the relationship? *Journal of Advanced Nursing*, **6(6)**, 491–6.

Delbecq, A., Van der Ven, A. H. and Gustafson, D. H. (1975). *Group Techniques for Programme Planning: a Guide to Nominal and Delphi Processes*. Scott, Foresman, Glenville.

Department of Health (1989a). *Working for Patients*, HMSO, London.

Department of Health. (1989b). *A Strategy for Nursing*. DoH, London.

Dickens, P. (1990). Aiming for excellence in mental handicap services. *International Journal of Health Care Quality Assurance*, **3(1)**, 4–8.

Dickoff, J. and James, P. (1968). A theory of theories: a position paper. *Nursing Research*, **17(3)**, 197–203.

Donabedian, A. (1966). Evaluating the quality of medical care. *Millbank Memorial Fund Quarterly*, **44(2)**, 166–206.

Donabedian, A. (1980). *Explorations in Quality Assessment and Monitoring. Volume 1. The Definition of Quality Assurance and Approaches to its Assessment*. Health Administration Press, Ann Arbor.

Donabedian, A. (1989). Institutional and professional responsibilities in quality assurance. *Quality Assurance in Health Care*, **1(1)**, 3–11.

Eriksen, L. R. (1987). Patient satisfaction: an indicator of nursing care quality? *Nursing Management*, **18(7)**, 31–5.

Fawcett, J. (1984). *Analysis and Evaluation of Conceptual Models of Nursing*. Davis, Philadelphia.

Fitzpatrick, J. J. (1989). The empirical approach to the development of nursing science. In *Conceptual Models of Nursing*, 2nd edn. J. J. Fitzpatrick and A. L. Whall (Eds), pp. 427–37. Appleton and Lange, Norwalk.

Goldstone, L. A., Ball, J. A. and Collier, M. M. (1984). *Monitor: An Index of the Quality of Nursing Care for Acute Medical and Surgical Wards*, Newcastle upon Tyne Polytechnic Products, Newcastle upon Tyne.

Hamric, A. B. (1989). A model for CNS evaluation In *The Clinical Nurse Specialist in Theory and Practice*. 2nd edn. A. B. Hamric, and J. A. Spross (Eds), pp. 83–104. Saunders, Philadelphia.

Handy, C. (1985). *Understanding Organizations*. 3rd edn. Penguin, Harmondsworth.

Hayward, J. (1975). *Information – a Prescription Against Pain*. Royal College of Nursing, London.

Healy, S. (1988). Health care quality assurance terminology. *International Journal of Health Care Quality Assurance*, **1(1)**, 20–32.

Hegyvary, S. T. and Haussmann R. K. D. (1976). Monitoring nursing care quality. *Journal of Nursing Administration*, **6(9)**, 3–9.

Hyde, P. (1984). Something for everyone. *Nursing Times*, **80(48)**, 49–50.

Keighley, T. (1989). Developments in quality assurance. *Senior Nurse*, **9(9)**, 7–10.

Kitson, A. and Kendall, H. (1986). Rest assured. *Nursing Times*, **82(35)**, 28–31.

Kitson, A. and Harvey, G. (1991). *Bibliography of Nursing Quality Assurance and Standards of Care 1932–1987*. Scutari, Harrow.

King's Fund. (1986). *Quality Circle Training Manual For Leaders and Facilitators*, King's Fund Centre, London.

Knaus, W. A., Draper, E. A., Wagner, D. P. and Zimmerman, J. E. (1986). An evaluation of outcome from intensive care in major medical centres. *Annals of Internal Medicine*, **104(3)**, 410–8.

Lancaster, J., and Lancaster, W. (Eds). (1982). *The Nurse as a Change Agent*. Mosby, St. Louis.

Lang, N. M. (1976). Issues in quality assurance in nursing. In *Issues in Evaluation Research*, American Nurses Association, pp. 45–6. ANA, Kansas City.

Lang, N. M. and Clinton, J. F. (1984a) *Quality assurance – the idea and its development in the United States*. In *Measuring the Quality of Care*. L. D. Willis and M. E. Linwood, (Eds), pp. 69–88. Churchill Livingstone, Edinburgh.

Lang, N. M. and Clinton, J. F. (1984b). Assessment of quality of nursing care. *Annual Review of Nursing Research*, **2**, 135–63.

Lees, J. and Dale, B. G. (1989). The use of quality circles in a health care environment. *International Journal of Health Care Quality Assurance*, **2(2)**, 5–12.

Leibold, S. (1983). Peer review. In *Clinical Nurse Specialist in Theory and Practice*. A. B. Hamric, and J. Spross. (Eds), pp. 219–33. Grune and Stratton, New York.

Lindblom, C. E. (1959). The science of muddling through. *Public Administration Review*, **19**, 79–88.

Lohr, K. N. (1988). Outcome measurement: concepts and questions. *Inquiry*, **25(1)**, 37–50.

Manley, K. (1990). Approach to gathering staff values and beliefs using a nominal group technique. Unpublished.

Manley, K. (1991a) A knowledge base for practice. In *Nursing: A Knowledge Base For Practice*. A. Perry and M. Jolley (Eds), pp. 1–27. Edward Arnold, London.

Manley, K. (1991b). Possible criteria and standards. Unpublished.

Manley, K. (1991c). Incremental goal orientated steps in the standard setting process. Unpublished.

Marek, K. (1989). Outcome measurement in nursing. *Journal of Nursing Quality Assurance*, **4(1)**, 1–9.

Maxwell, R. J. (1984). Quality assessment in health. *British Medical Journal*, **288**, 1470–2.

Miller, A. (1985). Nurse/patient dependency – is it iatrogenic? *Journal of Advanced Nursing*, **10(1)**, 63–9.

Morris, B. (1989). Total quality management. *International Journal of Health Care Quality Assurance*, **2(3)**, 4–6.

National Health Service Training Authority (1987). *Guide and Model Documentation for Individual Performance Review*. Rev. edn. NHSTA, Bristol.

Newcomb, K. A. and Kleiner, B. H. (1989). Managing for excellence in hospital institutions. *International Journal of Health Care Quality Assurance*, **2(3)**, 14–6.

Nightingale, F. (1859). *Notes on Nursing*, Harrison, London.

Open University, (1985). *Caring for Health: History and Diversity*. Open University Press, Milton Keynes.

Orem, D. E. (1985). *Nursing: Concepts of Practice*. 3rd edn. McGraw-Hill, New York.

Orlando, I. (1961). *The Dynamic Nurse-Patient Relationship*. Putman, New York.

Peplau, H. E. (1952). *Interpersonal Relations in Nursing*. Putman, New York.

Perrin, J. (1990). *Resource Management in the NHS*. Chapman & Hall, London.

Peters, T. J. and Austin, N. K. (1985). *A Passion for Excellence*. Random House, New York.

Peters, T. J. and Waterman, R. H. (1982). *In Search of Excellence: Lessons from America's Best-run Companies*. Harper & Row, New York.

Phaneuf, M. C. (1964). A nursing audit method. *Nursing Outlook*, **12(5)**, 42–5.

Ramphal, M. (1974) Peer review. *American Journal of Nursing*, **74(1)**, 63–7.

Riehl-Sisca, J. P. (1989). *Conceptual Models for Nursing Practice*, 3rd edn. Appleton & Lange, Norwalk.

Robinson, N. M. (1987). Directions in person-environment research in mental retardation, In *Living Environments and Mental Retardation*. S. Landesman, P. Vietze, and M. Beggab (Eds). American Association on Mental Retardation, Washington.

Robson, M. (1988). *Quality Circles: a Practical Guide*. Gower, Aldershot.

Rogers, M. E. (1989). Nursing: a science of unitary human beings, In *Conceptual Models for Nursing Practice*, 3rd edn, J. P. Riehl-Sisca (Ed), pp. 181–8. Appleton & Lange, Norwalk.

Roy, C. (1984). *Introduction to Nursing: an Adaptation Model*. 2nd Edn. Prentice-Hall, Englewood Cliffs.

Royal College of Nursing (1984). *Setting Standards of Nursing Care*. Unpublished draft. RCN, London.

Royal College of Nursing. (1990). *Quality Patient Care: the Dynamic Standard Setting System*. RCN, London.

Schön, D. A. (1983). *The Reflective Practitioner*. Basic Books, New York.

Schmadl, J. C. (1979). Quality assurance: examination of the concept. *Nursing Outlook*, **27(7)**, 462–5.

Shaw, C. D. (1986). *Introducing Quality Assurance*, King's Fund Centre, (King's Fund Project Paper No 64).

Shukla, R. K. (1981). Structure vs people in primary nursing: an enquiry. *Nursing Research*, **30(4)**, 236–41.

Smith-Marker, C. G. (1988) *Setting Standards for Professional Nursing: the Marker Model*, Resource Applications, Baltimore.

Spross, J. A. (1989). The CNS as collaborator. In *The Clinical Nurse specialist in Theory and Practice*. 2nd edn. A. B. Hamric and J. A. Spross (Eds), pp. 205–26. Saunders, Philadelphia.

Strong, P. and Robinson, J. (1988). *New Model Management: Griffiths and the NHS*, Nursing Policy Studies Centre, University of Warwick, Coventry.

Telford, W. A. (1979). *A Method of Determining Nursing Establishments*. The Author, Birmingham.

Van Maanen, H. M. (1979). Perspectives and problems on quality of nursing care: an overview of contributions from North America and recent developments in Europe. *Journal of Advanced Nursing*, **4(4)**, 377–89.

Van Maanen, H. M. (1981). Improvement of quality of nursing care: a goal to challenge in the eighties. *Journal of Advanced Nursing*, **6(1)**, 3–9.

Wandelt, M. and Ager, J. (1974). *Quality Patient Care Scale*. Appleton-Century-Crofts, New York.

Wandelt, M. and Stewart, D. S. (1975). *Slater Nursing Competencies Rating Scale*. Appleton-Century-Crofts, New York.

Warfield, C. and Manley, K. (1990). Developing a new philosophy in the NDU. *Nursing Standard*, **4(41)**, 27–30.

Waters, K. (1986). Cause and effect. *Nursing Times*, **82(5)**, 28–30.

Watkins, M. (1990). Nursing knowledge – ultimate objectives. In *Nursing: a Knowledge Base for Practice*. A. Perry and M. Jolley (Eds), pp. 308–42. Edward Arnold, London.

Wilson, C. R. M. (1987). *Hospital-Wide Quality Assurance*. Saunders, Toronto.

Wilson, J. and McNulty, L. (1991). *Resources for Practice*. Distance Learning Centre, South Bank Polytechnic, London.

Winch, A. E. (1989). Peer support and peer review. In *The Clinical Nurse Specialist in Theory and Practice*. 2nd edn. A. B. Hamric and J. A. Spross (Eds), Saunders, Philadelphia.

Wright, D. (1984). An introduction to the evaluation of nursing care: a review of the literature. *Journal of Advanced Nursing*, **9(5)**, 457–67.

8 Caring – a developing art: philosophical and spiritual reflections

All the major nurse theoreticians, who are concerned with the nature of man and the nature of the nurse in relationship to caring for the distressed, sick, fragile, immature or broken human individual, bring into the sphere of their concerns the welfare of the human spirit (Leinginger, 1981; Watson, 1985; Rogers, 1980; Parse, 1981). The human spirit is not easy to define, and perhaps there is an argument that could be successfully developed that suggests that the human spirit per definition is, humanly speaking, indescribable. That the human spirit is not of this 'world' is taken as a basic premise for any writing on spirituality, and thus any definitions of the spirit, the nature of human spirituality, and the essence of spiritual life, will use rather abstruse theological language that is inadequate for the task from its very foundations, and yet the best that the human mind can engender, to help clarify and compose thoughts on the subject. Nurse theoreticians speak of the human spirit in neoclassical terms, such as – 'that which inspires in one the desire to transcend the realm of the material' (Labun, 1988). Burnard (1990) adds that 'often the notion of a spirit is associated with the existence of God. The idea seems to be that the spirit of the person is the "God" aspect of them'. Additionally, most writers on spirituality in their definition of the spirit seem to include the notion of a search for meaning. As Burnard (1987) reflects:

> 'It would seem that the need to find meaning in what we do is a basic human need . . . Such meaning may be framed within the context of a set of religious beliefs that can take very varied forms . . .'

Labun (1988) points out that spiritual well-being is a form of total wholeness commenting that it is present

> 'when the person experiences wholeness within the self, with other human beings, and in transcendence with another realm. Spiritual integrity is demonstrated through acts that show qualities such as love, hope, trust and forgiveness.'

Such encompassing definitions and concepts of the spiritual and spirituality accommodate almost all viewpoints and philosophical outlooks. For the purpose of these reflections, spirituality will be defined according to Labun as

1. An aspect of the total person which is related to and integrated with the functioning and expression of all other aspects of the person';
2. A relational nature which is expressed through interpersonal relationships between persons and through a transcendent relationship with another realm';
3. Involving relationships and producing behaviours and feelings which demonstrate the existence of love, faith, hope and trust, therein providing meaning to life and a reason for being'.

(Labun, 1988)

Given this perception by nurses of the nature of the human spirit, it is not surprising that they also see spirituality from a particular perspective (Oliver, 1990). Only humans are capable of a conscious spiritual life, that is, only humans are aware that there is something more to their lives than biological, psycho-social or cultural realities; a perception that no other living creature possesses; an awareness that there is a 'spirit' of self, independent of, but fundamental to, a tangible bio-psycho-social self, where the latter can be more or less adequately analysed, understood and controlled; and the former, with much more difficulty, is a realisation that is not always couched in religious terminology (Parse, 1981; Rogers, 1980; Watson, 1985). Nurse theoreticians rarely talk of the human spirit and its concerns in the same way as they refer to the observations of religious practices, since it is more a psycho-social and cultural necessity to 'practicse' religious observances than a purely or distinctly spiritual need (Leininger, 1981; Watson, 1988; Labun, 1988). Nonetheless, there is a part of spirituality that calls for a minimum of 'religious' observances, in order that the observant practitioner of a religion may maintain a significant level of spiritual integrity (Burnard, 1987; Stoll, 1979; Beeny, 1990; Labun, 1988). Not all spiritual needs however are determined by religious observances; although all major religions attempt with varying success to satisfy the spiritual needs of their followers. When nurses refer to the spiritual nature of man, when they talk of the elemental spirituality of the individual, they are encompassing far more than just religious needs or religious activities (Labun, 1988; Burnard, 1987; Dugan, 1987–8; Oliver, 1990; Steeves and Kahn, 1987). If that were the case, atheists, agnostics, pantheists and naturalists, to list but a few categories of individuals, would be left without spiritual support. All individuals are seen as integrally consisting of spirit, mind and matter, including atheists, agnostics, pantheists and avowed socio-realists or secular humanists. The spirit referred to is not necessarily a recognis-able 'Christian', 'Jewish', 'Islamic' or 'Hindu' spirit, in communion with Christian, Jewish, Islamic or Hindu philosophy and religion. Rather, it is that aspect of the human nature that on the one hand differentiates humans from all other species of life and the unique individual human spirit from anyone else's, but also that very essence of self that unites the human individual with all of creation in a timeless manner and with all other human spirits. To the extent that the human spirit has the power to divide and separate while simultaneously to unite and hold together all of creation, it is a forceful entity far greater than any mere psycho-social and cultural force could ever be (Rogers, 1980; Watson, 1988; Parse, 1981). This is not to deny the value of psycho-social, cultural and religious forces in our lives, but to emphas-ise that spirituality, as it is defined by nurse-theoreticians and by most theologians, has more to do with eschatological realities and human transcendency than with Sunday observances or kosher diets (Dugan, 1987–88; Taylor and Ferszt, 1990; Steeves and Kahn, 1987; Kreidler, 1984). Eschatological realities are based on religious doctrines that concern the final and last events of a person's life, such as death, the last judgement, belief in an afterlife and concepts of heaven and hell. To the extent that an individual is religiously motivated in the expres-sion of their spirituality, to that extent eschatological doctrines may profoundly influence them.

The question to pursue now is 'why should nurses be concerned with human spirituality in such a particular manner?' Perhaps the most obvious reason is that since humans have a spirit which binds and holds together the very essence of their individuality and also unites them with all other humans, the nurse, who also has a spirit and is united to the patient or client as to another individual with a human spirit, the concern is potentially of human mutual interest (Mayeroff, 1971). The nurse is concerned and interested because she or he, also has a human spirit and the interest is on a 'peer' humanitarian and humane relation-ship level. There is also the professional rationale for interest in human spirituality, namely that nurses themselves, patients, clients and their friends and relations are all more likely to display spiritual distress in times of anxiety, sadness, fear and deep emotional and psychological trauma than at other times (McGlone, 1990; Dugan, 1987–88; Bur-nard, 1987). It is precisely when the human spirit is rendered most vulnerable and fragile by infirmity, disease, major change in lifestyle or physical and/or psychological trauma that the nurse is most likely to meet the 'wounded soul' (Watson, 1985; Leininger, 1981).

If nurse theoreticians claim that the nurse should be concerned with the *whole* human person, not just his physical being, and they indeed maintain that the human individual is far more complex and forceful than any combination of his 'constituent parts', of which the human spirit is the motivator, animator and binder of the human personality, then the nurse should rightfully be interested in human spirituality, be concerned specifically about his or her own human spirit and how this interacts with the human spirit of her patient (Rogers, 1980; Leininger, 1981; Watson, 1985; Watson, 1988; Parse, 1981; Parse, 1989). The nurse is concerned about spirituality because this is part of her patients' nature of being. The patient is additionally more likely to draw the attention of the nurse to himself, because his spirit's equilibrium is affected by the presence of disease, distress, trauma or anxiety. The patient may display signs of spiritual distress and the nurse practising holistic nursing may wish to intervene and, according to many writers, ought to intervene (Rogers, 1980; Leininger, 1981; Aamodt, 1988; Liehr, 1989).

Nurses, as all health-care professionals, have a tendency to intervene at the slightest indication of a patient's dis-equilibrium. This meddling approach can be shrugged off as beginner's over zealousness or it can be seen as a more deep-seated evidence of the nurse's own distress and inadequate coping mechanisms (Speck, 1988). T. S. Eliot, in the timeless manner of poets, begs God to 'teach us to care and not to care' (Eliot, 1963), since an interfering, meddle-some caring can be as devastating as 'no caring at all'. Spiritual distress is as unique to an individual as is their own spirit, therefore, at the core of spiritual distress is a profound loneliness that cannot ever be reached by another human individual (Bakan, 1968; Evely, 1967). Edna St Vincent Millay, writing about her inability to hear a friendly voice in her loneliness, woefully points out, 'and I listened for a voice; – but my heart was all I heard, . . . ' when she was 'searching (her) heart for its true sorrow' (St V. Millay, 1964).

Spiritual distress and spiritual pain, like physical, cultural and psychological pain is an utterly lonely experience (Bakan, 1968), yet paradoxically it is the very manifestation of such distress that is the person's opportunity not only to cry for help but also to start returning to the fellowship of other humans from their self appointed exile of inner disharmony (Bakan, 1968; Evely, 1967; Speck, 1988). As Bakan points out 'pain is also a means of returning to the dominion of the social telos' (Bakan, 1968). Spiritual pain has the added poignancy that it often centres around transcendental and eschatological issues of life, death, vulnerability and guilt. The afflicted individual is likely to concur with the Greek chorus in Sophocles' ageless tragedy, Antigone, that 'happy are they who know not the taste of evil', because surely 'from a house that heaven hath shaken the curse departs not' (Sophocles, 1947). This conviction of humans down the ages that invariably we are to blame for our life events and life processes, including illnesses, disease and misfortune, results in our desperate search for meaning and rationale in apparently senseless, motiveless or inexplicable tragedies that confront us, for as in the times of Sophocles so today, 'this law is immutable for mortals greatly to live is greatly to suffer'

(Sophocles, 1947). The search for the meaning of suffering and the essence of life and self is what fuels the loneliness of spiritual distress. Dugan, in his analysis of three indicators of spiritual distress, lists loss of meaning as one of the elementary ingredients in spiritual disequilibrium (Dugan, 1987–88). Likewise, Speck, in his monograph on 'pastoral care in time of illness', reflects that one of the signs or indicators of spiritual distress is loss of meaning in life, a sense of meaninglessness and hopelessness (Speck, 1988).

Kreidler, in a beautifully presented reflection on the need for nurses to develop their own philosophies of life, and urging them to find meaning in their lives in order to be in a better position to work with distressed patients, wryly observed that all too often 'faced with the overwhelming reality of suffering, nurses cope with their own feelings of inadequacy by distancing themselves from patients' (Kreidler, 1984). This she claims is partly due to a lack of understanding by nurses, that both their own searching for meaning in suffering and the patient's search is something natural, positive and growth enducing, and not a sign of weakness. Thus she continues:

> 'Nurses need assurance that groping for meaning in suffering is not a sign of deep-seated neurosis, but rather a sign of strength . . . Our spiritual distress when facing suffering must be explored and understood if we are to be able to minister to our patients' needs.'
> (Kreidler, 1984)

It is the poet, however, who reminds us that searching for meaning in life is above all natural:

> 'Sorrow's springs are the same. Nor mouth had, no nor mind expressed what heart heard of, ghost guessed: It is the blight man was born for.'
> (Hopkins, 1964)

The suffering servant who is spiritually smitten not only physically and psychologically is a constant theme in Judaeo-Christian writings and expressed nowhere so eloquently as in the trans-cultural and transcendental biblical writings of the authors of the Book of Job. Job, the suffering Innocent, eloquently describes his torments as:

> 'My days die away like an echo;
> My heart-strings are snapped.'

and the would-be biblical nurse is faced with controlling an unconsolable spirit, for how is the nurse to fix 'snapped heart-strings'? (Habel, 1975). Job explains the source of his woes, like Sophocles' Antigone:

> 'Pity me, pity me, you that are my friends; for the hand of God has touched me'.

> (Sophocles, 1947)

and yet Job sees no remedy from the consequences of being touched by God. He *wants* solely pity or perhaps, using today's vocabulary, we would talk about compassion, or an empathetic presence, for he sees no other source of help. He rightfully queries how can anyone intervene and console him? Job describes the pangs of his anguish:

> 'When I stop to think, I am filled with horror, and my whole body is convulsed'.

Many a time the nurse or friend watches apparently helplessly as the afflicted person is literally convulsed at the horror and thought of their loneliness and desolation; nonetheless the presence of another is felt, and at some level appreciated and considered to be necessary by those spiritually smitten (BK). The often repeated phrase 'to have the patience of Job' refers not so much to Job's apparently resigned passivity; Job was anything but passive about his sad state of afflictions, but to his inner strength and above all patient endurance. Although Job did not perceive himself as having much inner strength, it was precisely in his innermost being where he perceived himself to be most alone and abandoned (in human terms) that he was most akin to Him, of whom he was the patriarchal precursor. Job at the time does not see this; he laments:

> 'Have I the strength to wait?
> What end have I to expect, that I
> should be patient?
> Is my strength the strength of stone,
> or is my flesh bronze?
> Oh how shall I find help within myself?
> The power to aid myself is put out of my reach.'

The nurse is advised to simply listen to the patient or client, and *be there*, as an 'unintruding but forceful presence understanding that few words or actions of themselves can ameliorate the situation'. The companionship of accompanying the patient on a difficult journey is an analogy brought out by several writers (Campbell, 1984; Campbell, 1985; Speck, 1988). This may be because in spiritual distress the spirit of the patient is struggling with God Himself (or some form of Transcendency) and no human intervention could be of any use here. Evely explains the case as if 'the weight of your unhappiness crushes you, but against God, to the point of not leaving any space between Him and you' (Evely, 1967). Bakan adds that 'physical and spiritual pain are among the most salient of human experiences; and it often precipitates questioning the meaning of life itself' (Bakan, 1968).

If this were the case, can or should any human wedge the two apart? Would it be truly therapeutic to disrupt this process? Evely goes on to say that since it is in 'darkness and effort that we find usefulness and value'; and that pain and suffering, especially spiritual suffering, tends to make one 'revolt against the universe, to lose one's place and one's rights in it, to become vulnerable over the whole extent of one's being'.

It would appear that what Evely is arguing for is permission for the 'afflicted person' to *feel* his spiritual pain, so as to be subsequently able to truly understand what is important and central (Evely, 1967). Rather than advocating avoidance of spiritual distress, perhaps we should be looking at ways of demonstrating our fellowship, presence and support for those experiencing such a state of disequilibrium, by acknowledging the precious nature of the distress (Burnard, 1987; Labun, 1988). The patient needs to be supported and reminded that he is not unusual or bizarre, for 'there is a prodigious fraternity in the human condition: everybody gasps under a weight which he is incapable of bearing' (Evely, 1967).

The distraught patient, who is now confronted with a painful spiritual process, which they themselves often attribute to the consequences of their lives, since they have 'gone *their* way, to the outermost limit of daring and have stumbled against Law enthroned' (Sophocles, 1947). They may be ready to acknowledge their spiritual distress, working through perceived guilt and sorting out relationships with themselves, their family and friends and ultimately with matters of the Spirit. This is a necessary and unavoidable consequence of being human (Stoll, 1979; McGlone, 1990; Taylor and Ferszt, 1990; Watson, 1988; Gaylin, 1985). As the Greeks so eloquently phrased it, they are being 'touched by the hand of God' (Sophocles, 1947).

The manifestations of being 'touched by the hand of God' are not, however, uniform phenomena. Although the poet may class all such occurrences as 'wrestling with my God' (Hopkins, 1953), the careful observer may indeed differentiate between the types of spiritual disequilibrium that are presented. Thus, Labun in a fascinating article looking into the need for more thorough assessments of a patient's spiritual wellbeing, as part of a nurse's total holistic nursing approach to patient care, lists seven possible states of spiritual integrity, namely, spiritual pain, alienation, anxiety, guilt, anger, loss and despair (Labun, 1988). Needless to say these states may come singly, overlap, or be part of an ongoing process; and the individual may move back and forth between the states for quite a while. Again it is the religious poet who best sums up the entire field of experience, crying:

'O the mind, mind has mountains; cliffs of fall
Frightful, sheer, no-man-fathomed. Hold them cheap

May who ne'er hung there. Nor does long small our
Durance deal with that steep or deep.'

(Hopkins, 1953)

What then, is the role of a nurse in demonstrating caring behaviours towards a patient who not only is in psycho-social and physical discomfort and pain (hence in contact with the health-care services), but also in spiritual distress – a situation not all that infrequent? How does one care in a situation like this? Edna St Vincent Millay, describing a woman in just such a situation, said

> 'She had a look about her that I wish I could forget – the look of a scared thing, sitting in a net!'

(St V. Millay, 1964)

This image of the frail wounded bird is quite frequent and one that a nurse can identify with reasonably easily. Sometimes the person in spiritual distress appears belligerent and angry and it is hard to see past this exterior mask. All too often, in instances like these, the nurse will assume the presence of a degree of psychological distress, but not think that spiritual disintegration lies at the bottom of the pain and sorrow, manifested so loudly and brusquely (Labun, 1986; Heron, 1989; Dugan, 1987–88). There is a tendency to imagine that the patient in predominantly spiritual distress will have the persona of the 'wounded animal' but this certainly is not always the case, and indeed may be just a phase in a series of stages from disintegration to spiritual re-affirmation of self in respect of God, the Universe, others and one's own inner private being. Certainly not infrequently spiritual distress is confused with depression or psychological instability. Gaylin, in a provocative essay on 'Feelings', stated the often forgotten truism that:

> ' . . . feelings are internal directives essential for human life. In addition and not just in passing, they are their own rewards. They are the means *and* the ends.'

(Gaylin, 1985)

The patient in spiritual distress, displaying a whole array of emotions ranging through fear, bewilderment, anguish, loneliness, but also anger and dissatisfaction, to name but a few, is not only thereby stating that he is fully human and is capable of these emotions, but is also crying for all that is left to him like Job, i.e. human contact, human connectedness (Labun, 1988).

Gaylin continues in describing the functions of emotions by stating:

> 'Emotions then are not just directives to ourselves but directives from others to us, indicating that we have been seen, that we have

been understood, that we have been appreciated, that we have made contact.'

We are all capable of displaying feelings, and manifestations of feelings have a role to play in transmitting our innermost thoughts and states:

> 'even without knowing why, we respond to the feelings of others. Emotions are contagious.'
>
> (Gaylin, 1985)

It now becomes clearer why correct interpretation of emotions becomes crucial in the instance of spiritual distress among patients, for in psycho-social distress, perhaps advice, health-education, counselling or active intervention in the social sphere of a patient's life, may be necessary. In spiritual distress, however, the single most efficacious act on the part of a nurse may be a quiet presence (Burnard, 1967; Labun, 1988; McGlone, 1990). Intervention, in the sense of actively doing something for, with or to the patient, becomes meaningless here, for the nature of the distress is a particular form of pain which is utterly lonely. The pains are suffered in loneliness, thoughts left unvoiced 'to hoard unheard, heard unheeded' (Hopkins, 1953). Indeed one is not aiming here at necessarily reducing the pain or even its perception, but attempting to facilitate the patient's passing through the crises (Labun, 1988; Burnard, 1987). In order to be able to do that adequately, the nurse herself needs to feel comfortable and in control of her own life and its meaning, at least sufficiently not to be overwhelmed by the anguish and sorrow of the patient (Kreidler, 1984). As Kreidler points out:

> 'Nurses can become overwhelmed by suffering to which they cannot relate or which causes them to feel helpless, inadequate or guilty . . . A clear need is expressed by nurses, patients and researchers for some approach which will aid the nurse who feels distress when dealing with those who suffer.'
>
> (Kreidler, 1984)

Although working through such issues is possible in a totally non-religious context and some nurse theoreticians would appear to be suggesting that this is possible (Leininger, 1981; Watson, 1985; Rogers, 1980), for the religiously minded patient in spiritual distress, the nurse too may need to share (or at least to be open to) some of the religious constructs of the patient's world (Taylor and Ferszt, 1990; McGlone, 1990; Beeny, 1990; Robbins, 1991). Such knowledge of various faith traditions is not likely to occur with every patient, and some people in need of spiritual caring will only admit to their inner world of pain and anguish to selected people, who may or may not be of the same spiritual inclination, religious observance, or socio-cultural grouping. It is also stated that meaning in suffering may be found in a particular religious context, as Kreidler notes:

> 'It may be gleaned through a "leap of faith" which says that there is no meaning to be found other than that which is beyond one's self; that which transcends man's ability to know that which is God.'
>
> (Kreidler, 1984)

There is therefore a legitimate doubt, and room for questioning, whether one should advocate that the nurse should be prepared to cater for every patient's spiritual needs, and be concerned about 'caring for the spirit of all her patients.' This rather obvious observation, however, does not integrate well with the basic tenets of caring theories and somehow the solicitous nurse intuitively realises that she should be concerned with the whole patient, which would include awareness of a spiritual dimension to the human individual, and therefore also address that area of a patient's being (Leininger, 1981; Watson, 1985; Rogers, 1980). It could be suggested therefore that nurses need to be at least minimally aware of the spiritual dimension of a patient's life and of the spiritual dimensions of their own lives, for 'meaning in life is never predetermined. It is discovered by each person in his own living' (Kreidler, 1984). This awareness and insight will more likely then, coupled with better communication skills, enable the nurse to determine the required level of caring-healing intervention required when confronted with a patient who appears to be in spiritual distress (Watson, 1985; Burnard, 1987; Labun, 1988). It would be presumptuous and against the essence of human spirituality to suggest that every or any nurse can address the spiritual pain of any or every patient. Part of the mystery of the pain lies in its intensely individualistic character and specifically non-categorisable nature; the very best a nurse can do is acknowledge its presence, and help the patient *confront* the spiritual issues raised.

Committed presence

Acknowledging the presence of spiritual pain in a patient and helping them move through the critical episode can take several forms (Labun, 1988; Dugan, 1987–88). Certainly being with a patient is not just a matter of sitting down next to a patient. Consider the familiar scene of the inadequately prepared agency or relief nurse who is called in to perform a 'special duty' in a medical ward, for a patient who is recovering from a suicide attempt. The patient is desolate, dejected, utterly alone with himself and his thoughts, and confused, in need of gentle peace and loving re-assurance, if not immediate moves at re-integration into human society. This entirely lonely patient is now confronted with an 'alien' soul, sitting too close to him for 'allowed' social contact and therefore violating the usual cultural norms of our society – and usually engrossed in a newspaper held open sufficiently wide so as to cover the face. The nurse is thus 'too close' for comfort, but entirely *absent* from any level of meaningful human contact. The patient is initially surprised, then dismayed and all too often, subsequently, angry and left feeling insulted and even more unwanted and disregarded. How much more hurting can it be for a confused desperately lonely person, who has seriously contemplated removing himself from human society precisely because he does not see himself in it, to be faced with a member of a caring profession, whose sole purpose of 'presence' appears to be the fulfillment of custodial duties; thereby removing the last vestige of self-control the person has left, i.e. to choose to live or not to live!

It is not the author's purpose here to debate the rationale for or mechanisms of treatment plans for patients suffering from depression or post-suicidal anxieties. Rather the example is used to demonstrate that in an instance where the human spirit, not only the psyche, is most evidently and profoundly wounded and in need of healing (which bears little correlation to actual level of physical self-inflicted harm), the apparently accepted form of nursing response is to send to such a spiritually desolate person an often inadequately qualified professional, who is to protect the patient from further *physical* self-harm, while in the process, most evidently, ignoring the spiritual and psychological needs of the patient.

Physical close presence of the nurse is observed, but the nurse is not present to the patient. She is not present to the patient, for she has not and perhaps intends not to establish contact or ties with him. One of the hardest skills to learn is the skill of therapeutic quiet, active presence, especially in the context of a short professional relationship, a presence that can be best described as 'committed presence'.

Speck would place the role of the hospital chaplain, hopefully the expert facilitator in matters of spiritual growth and spirituality, firmly in the realm of a committed, quiet, enabling Presence (Speck, 1988). Citing Potter's play *Singing Detective*, he also adds to the legion of examples of what a truly committed spiritual presence should *not* be. He says that the over-zealous evangelising health-care worker who invades wards and encourages the sick to take hymn-sheets so that 'you'll be able to follow – please take one!', is, according to him, simply imposing his religiosity and specific brand of religion on the most spiritually vulnerable (Speck, 1988). These patients are broken, devastated and frightened ill people, not free to move away from the pious onslaughts of some members of the general public.

The ethical implications of such an approach to spirituality are highly questionable. These evangelical proselytisers are inevitably inviting the classic response of one of Potter's more outspoken patients: 'Leave us alone! Why don't you bugger off and leave us in peace . . .' (Speck, 1988). Communal acts of worship have a part to play in hospital life but should not be imposed on patients; any more than impromptu ward-wide hymn-singing or encouraging group recitation of the rosary!

Committed presence involves some aspects of counselling, but mostly it involves sharing one's own commitment to life and to the other, by means of physical and spiritual presence *to* the patient (Watson, 1985; Labun, 1988; Kreidler, 1984). This quiet often silent presence may involve time. It certainly can involve an element of 'taming'. The patient in spiritual distress may find it only possible to 'open-up' to his God or his Comforter. Human intervention here, at least initially, would be misguided. The role of the nurse may be, however, simply to allow and create for the patient the 'space' to work through the spiritual issues confronting him (Burnard, 1987; Labun, 1988). The nurse may monitor the situation and gently determine whether there is someone that the patient would like to share thoughts with or something that he would like done, e.g. to arrange to receive a sacrament, read a spiritual book or even look at a religious programme on television. Often patients are embarrassed to ask for these services outright, although they are quite entitled to enquire after them. They are embarrassed not so much out of diffidence towards nurses, but because spiritual matters are perceived to be the last bastion of privacy; to talk about spiritual matters is considered impolite or at least anti-social, and the whole area of spirituality is shrouded in an aura of unspeakable 'taboo'.

Human sexuality and aspects of dying are considered ultimate taboos by health-care workers and the public since their reality, especially in a hospital environment, is constantly being flouted most ignobly; but spirituality is the aspect of human existence which is virtually unexplored by health-care workers! The spiritual 'taming', therefore, that a health-care worker may need to practise, is that level of 'accompaniment' required to enable a client or patient to acknowledge his own need for spiritual help, be it self-engendered spiritual help or with the assistance of another kindred spirit, such as a chaplain (Speck, 1988; Campbell, 1988).

When Saint Exupery's Little Prince asked the fox what he meant by 'taming', the fox replied: 'It is an act too often neglected. It means to establish ties'. (Saint Exupery, 1974). He goes on to explain ties as a form of mutual, reciprocal needing, one of the other; . . . 'if you tame me, then we shall need each other. To me, you will be unique in all the world. To you I shall be unique in all the world . . .' (Saint Exupery, 1974). The nurse needs to convince the patient that he is unique, that he does matter, that nothing about him will alter that specialness, and that the spiritual dimension of life is also vitally important to her.

This process of convincing, this display of what Campbell refers to as 'moderated love' is what the little fox calls 'taming' (Campbell, 1988). Mayeroff in his book *On Caring* also refers quite a bit to the need for humans *to care and be cared for*; for to enable caring to occur is to allow oneself to be cared for. This self-caring occurs primarily on a personal individualistic level and then by others. Only when we learn to care for ourselves and learn to let others care for us is it possible to thera-peutically reach out and start to care for strangers. This, according to Mayeroff, enables growth to occur and for true growth to occur, a form of mutual taming is required (Mayeroff, 1971). The nurse as much as the patient must allow herself to be tamed and the patient as much as the nurse must trust that the taming is genuine and honest. Honesty is in fact one of Mayeroff's eight caring constructs, and it is also included in Leininger and Watson's work (Mayeroff, 1971; Watson, 1985; Leininger, 1981).

True caring involves growth, mutual growth of the carer and cared for, and it is this ability to grow, to change, to progress from pain and distintegration to purpose and equilibrium that gives the caring phe-nomena its impetus and rationale (Mayeroff, 1971; Kreidler, 1984; Watson, 1985). Allowing and creating an atmosphere in which the patient can develop 'ties', and can be tamed, for the purpose of inner healing, is certainly not easy and involves the taking of risks. It also carries with it the seeds of the next problem, that of the pain of parting, of separating, of growing away, for as Saint Exupery's little fox concludes:

'You become responsible, forever, for what you have tamed.'
(Saint Exupery, 1974)

The mutual opening up and taming of nurse and patient is therefore central to the caring-healing act and results in mutual growth. In fact, it is the evidence of mutual growth that reassures the parties that caring has occured (Watson, 1985; Mayeroff, 1971). Caring, evidenced by growth, is needed if the spirit is to be healed. Nurse theoreticians regard healing as one of the chief measurable outcomes of caring. When caring occurs, there is restoration of equilibrium, spiritual and psychological distress abates and growth can take place. It is growth and the growing potential that characterises healing (Rogers, 1980; Watson, 1985; Heron, 1989).

Touch

Committed presence can also include an element of touching the patient. Whereas in committed presence the nurse need not be with the patient all of the time, but her presence is still *felt* by the patient, who is convinced that the nurse though off duty or engaged elsewhere on the ward, is still concerned as much in her absence as when she is physically present with the patient; obviously the benefits of physically *touching* the patient are circumscribed to those moments of physical presence.

Psychologists and social anthropologists, and lately nurses and nurse-anthropologists studying caring constructs, have all commented on the profound significance of touch in the range of emotional responses available to the human individual (Pratt and Mason, 1981; Montague, 1971; Leininger, 1981; Bergman, 1983). Many animals, most mammals and all higher primates use various forms of touch to display emotions and felt wants, and touch in turn appears to fulfil many basic primitive needs (Montagu, 1971; Pratt and Mason 1981). It appears that humans need to be touched to develop normally (Montagu, 1971). Touch is part of the basic requirement for normal psycho-social growth and development, and many subsequent psychological maladjustments can be traced to inadequate physical caring in infancy, such as lack of sufficient touch, by fondling, cuddling, rocking and feeding. This may be due to primary physiological reasons, such as immaturity, congenital deformity, illness necessitating isolation, and so on. The importance of touch for the developing child cannot be over-emphasised. What is less clear is the continued value of touch for the adult.

Some popular psychologists and anthropologists like Rollo May, Clark, Moustakas or Montagu, advocate the need for more sustained meaningful touching into and through adult life, especially in times of distress (May, 1977; Moustakas, 1975; Montagu, 1971; Pratt and Mason, 1981). The wounded human psyche, experiencing spiritual distress and loneliness can only manifest its anxiety verbally and/or in some form of body language. The inherent nature of spiritual distress precludes much verbal interaction or use of linguistic intervention, but leaves much scope for non-verbal intervention, especially in the form of physical touch (Speck, 1988; Taylor and Ferszt, 1990).

Nurses and carers touch patients and relatives a lot, mostly during the course of performing specific nursing actions. The touch required to demonstrate caring behaviours is its own primary goal, it is not secondary to some other nursing function. However, the professional nurse holding a patient's hand may well at the same time assess for skin texture, warmth, presence of moisture or even muscle strength, as in the case of suspected stroke or shock or suspected presence of physical as well as psycho-spiritual pain. The nurse may gently touch the hand or hold the hand or hands of someone distressed, but the permission to do this must come directly from the patient, either by tacit approval or by overt request, such as 'Nurse, please hold me, I'm so afraid', or 'don't let me go', 'don't leave me alone', and so on. If a patient trusts the nurse sufficiently to admit to the presence of spiritual distress, he often also trusts sufficiently to allow the nurse to physically share his private space.

It is well to remember that purposefully touching someone is a very intrusive act, entirely invading an individual's private space. Nurses often intuitively take hold of a patient's hand, indicating by this action concern and willingness to share and lighten the patient's emotional burden. Taking hold of a patient's hand often takes place while the nurse or the patient is talking, but it can also take the place of verbal interaction. A nurse may also cradle or hug a patient, and by this non-verbal interaction convey far more than words are normally capable of doing. Rebecca Bergman, in her sensitive article on the nature of empathetic touch, cites the example of a nurse who 'broke through' a patient's isolation and distress by non-ceremoniously, intuitively embracing an old lady and cradling her in her arms. The woman felt she 'belonged' again and her pain abated (Bergman, 1983). For the lonely, bewildered, frightened patient, wrestling with issues of life and death in spiritual and psychological torment, subjection of self to being cradled or hugged is the supreme admission of total disintegration, hence this child-like stance towards the parent-figure means that ironically most poignantly links him or her with the rest of the suffering adult human race. It is mature self-awareness and recognition of personal distress that allows the adult patient to submit to such intimate loving touch and allow healing of the spirit to commence, (Moustakas, 1975). The nurse who is sitting on the patient's bed and spontaneously leans over to hug the patient as she observes the patient's eyes fill up with tears and the lips start to tremble is as much manifesting caring behaviours as the nurse who quietly listens to a patient re-tell his story of woes and tribulations. Likewise, the paediatric nurse who cradles the young parentless child to sleep is anaesthetising a pain, fortunately long-forgotten by most adults. One nursing instructor recalling her childhood stay in hospital, commented once to the author, 'I thought my mother had stopped loving me, that is why she left me alone in the hospital'. The intensity of such childhood pains is sometimes recalled however by adults, as they face new psychological and spiritual trauma and then again they feel totally alone and hurting, as they did in their childhood. The pain is renewed and the wound re-opened. Indeed, fortunate is the adult who has a faith life strong enough to carry them through such spiritual and psychological distress and anxiety.

Purposeful healing

Touch can also be manifest in such actions as caressing a person, squeezing a hand, giving someone a backrub or massage, even hair-washing, bed-bathing or tub-washing a patient, where the primary intention is manifestation of human purposeful, physical contact, more than secondary gains from increased circulation, cleanliness, freshness or increased muscle tone. Such actions as washing a patient's hair, where the real object is to make the patient feel good about themselves and raise their self-esteem, rather than maintaining personal hygiene, is primarily addressing the psycho-spiritual needs of a depressed patient.

In Benner's classic work, *From Novice to Expert*, she cites the example of a nurse who gave a rather sullen patient a backrub. Benner, observing the interaction, asked the nurse who was giving the backrub, whether it was considered a routine nursing procedure for her to do such an action. 'Yes,' she said, 'They found a lot of cancer, and he's in a pretty bad shape, but he doesn't talk about his feelings much. I like to use the backrub as a chance to talk to him and *as a different way of communicating with him.*' (Benner, 1984; emphasis mine).

Touch can also have profound and singular importance among certain categories of patients, such as those suffering from some specific sensory loss, such as sight or hearing, or those suffering from a contagious disease, trauma or disfiguring condition. Again, Brenner cites the example of two Accident and Emergency nurses, who realising that a patient was deaf, and seeing her in tears ('. . . you'd see the tears coming down her face . . . '), held her hand and kept repeating to her 'Everything is under control'. 'You just felt that was one of the most important things to do. Because she needed someone and she could only receive comfort and caring through touch and sight.' (Benner, 1984). The spiritual and psychological care evident here is indeed exemplary and Benner considered these nurses as manifesting 'expert' nursing judgements.

Nurses too use deliberate touch with patients that may be considered (usually wrongly) to have highly contagious diseases. For example, the author herself working with patients suffering from Hansen's Disease, even in the early days of her practice, never wore protective gloves when doing dressing changes, even though it was considered common medico-nursing practice at the time. The disease, however, was considered by *expert* epidemiologists to be minimally transmitted by social touching and direct physical touch for the lepromatous patient was extremely important for the patient's spiritual and psychological well-being. Indeed direct physical interaction with the patients was precisely practised to dismiss the notion of stigmatisation.

The inordinate sadness and loneliness conveyed in Betty Martin's title of her autobiographical book about life with Hansen's disease, '*No-one must ever know*', should have encouraged nurses even then to be more prepared to therapeutically and wisely use physical contact when at all possible. In this instance it was my informed intuition that guided my practice, more than the currently accepted nursing norm of the time.

The current situation with AIDS patients, closely mirrors these concerns and physical touch is considered an accepted way of showing to these patients love, concern and acceptance. No patient should ever have to feel they have a disease so easily transmittablc or 'awful' that work with such a patient precludes casual or even deliberate touch, as in holding a hand or caressing a child's head.

This position raises serious problems when nursing some patients with highly contagious diseases such as Lassa Fever or those with severe immunological disorders nursed in 'bubbles' and kept apart from normal, direct physical contact. A patient normally should not be denied this basic human caring action; for withholding human physical contact can have very serious subsequent consequences. It is Benner who, summarising the significance of expert nurses using touch therapeutically, adds ' . . . touch conveys relational and support messages as well as physical stimulation and comfort. It is perhaps symbolic of the direct laying on of hands, so central to nursing care. But touch, like any other form of communication, has many messages and must be used with discretion' (Benner, 1984).

Therapeutic attentive listening

Apart from committed presence and purposeful touch, there is also the skill of attentive healing listening. When the nurse is present with a patient, he may or may not be ready or prepared to talk, but the patient's anguish and torment may be quite evident to the nurse. It is appropriate here to simply be therapeutically present. Likewise not all patients can cry or demonstrate the depth of their distress, or if they do, it is more often when they are alone, often only asking for help and support once they begin to feel better, and therefore are more in control of their emotions and thoughts and in a stronger position to share concerns with strangers. This is not an unusual pattern of behaviour.

There is also the patient who manifests his distress and anxiety by talking about his spiritual state and here attentive healing listening is extremely important. The tone of voice, facial expression, patient's body language and choice of words all collude together to tell a story that is unique for that suffering patient. Attentive listening by the nurse helps the patient by allowing him to verbalise his concerns and to start addressing the crucial issues (Labun, 1988; Burnard, 1990; Taylor and Ferszt, 1990). By sharing thoughts and re-affirming their basic human origins which affect the spirit and human psyche, the 'lonely' patient can start to be re-integrated into society. In demonstrating a willingness to listen, the nurse shows concern and manifests her conviction that the patient's troubles are indeed significant and worthy of being listened to.

It is interesting to note that listening is one of the more often cited attributes of caring that nurses see themselves as employing. This attentive listening is not the work of junior staff nurses, as it is a very difficult skill to learn (Leininger, 1981; Watson, 1985; Rogers, 1980; Labun, 1988; Burnard, 1990). Often the patient will not spontaneously repeat himself so it is important to note what and how the patient recounts his tale first time round.

Although throughout this work there is talk of 'the patient', obviously in some instances the distress and spiritual anguish may be more manifested or more significantly evident among relatives and friends than by the senile or unconscious or paediatric patient. The attentive therapeutic listening may be directed in such cases to friends and relatives, who in addition to their own spiritual and psychological anguish at seeing their friend or relative suffer may also have reason to feel guilty, rightly or wrongly, or somewhat blameworthy of the patient's current predicament. The parent who ran over and killed his own toddler when backing out of the driveway on the day he was to move into a new larger council flat, only to be faced with accusing officials who told him that the flat was no longer his since he was now classed as 'childless', experiences spiritual torment that few young, nurses can easily appreciate.

This same father, a few years later, again found himself rushing his youngest child to hospital, to be told that the child was unconscious, needing intensive care and suffering from an inoperable brain-stem tumour. The spiritual distress of the child's parents and older sibling were understandably indescribable. The extent of the growth producing anguish experienced by the family was made clearer to the primary nurse who, knowing that they were nominally classed as practising Jews, observed 'I think I would have lost my faith, if it were me who had to go through this hell', to which the father responded 'It was only when we had lost absolutely everything, house, children, job, love and respect of society, that we realised we were alive and yet still had each other'. A response echoed so familiarly from the Book of Job. The absolute frankness and honesty of that response touched the nurse profoundly. Later that day, while the nurse was changing connecting tubes to the ventilator, the mother, almost in passing, said, 'It's really difficult; I'm all right when I'm here and I watch you, because I know you love Jamie a lot and I trust you. But when I go home I am violently sick every night. I can't keep anything down'.

The psychological cost of the stress the trauma had produced for the family was, using Evely's definition, 'unbearable', but out of that unspeakable double horror came a spiritual growth rarely witnessed. That couple, after the death of their second child, went on to help set up a self-help group for parents with children in paediatric intensive care units, and started to lecture up and down the country to parent groups and nursing students about the problems parents encounter in hospitals, intensive care units and in relation to public officials in times of stress and spiritual disintegration. It is also true, however, that at the time of Jamie's admission to the Intensive Care Unit the level of anguish that the parents were experiencing was not that obvious to the nursing staff.

That casual comment to the nurse put many other, otherwise insignificant, comments and actions into perspective. The parents in fact chose to confide in two fairly junior staff nurses, who though proficient paediatric nurses were not certified intensive care nurses. What the parents said they liked about those two nurses was their openness to their suggestions as to how care could best be delivered due to attentive listening. They often commented that they thought the two nurses were gentle with Jamie and cared more. This demonstration of preferences among parents for particular nursing staff is not uncommon and should be respected as much as possible, since it would be odd if someone could claim to like all nurses equally well, all of the time. To have natural preferences is human and to respect this as much as is equitable and possible is also a demonstration by nursing staff of reciprocal caring and love, if not respect for the parents' sorrow and unspoken grief.

Speck in his book *Being There* also recounts a similar case, where attentive therapeutic listening helped him, as the hospital chaplain, to minister to the needs of a distraught father who, having just given his adolescent daughter a moped, was now watching her die in an intensive care unit, after a lorry had knocked her down only hours after receiving the new gift. The father was blaming himself and projected his spiritual anguish upon the hapless clergyman. He wanted, indeed demanded, a miracle re his daughter's life, shouting, 'I also teach swimming to kids and, over the years, I've saved a few lives. Well . . . I reckon this time God owes me a life. You're a vicar, and you're going to get it for me. I need a miracle, so get down on your knees – and do it now!' (Speck, 1988). After the father had finished shouting and hitting out, he collapsed on the floor. The chaplain ' . . . joined him crouched on the floor (head to head, with his hand on his shoulder) and, after a while, again asked the father to tell him about his daughter; what sort of girl was she, what had happened that day. Gradually and painfully the story emerged' (Speck, 1988).

In this scenario the attentive therapeutic listening was accompanied by great sensitivity. By literally reaching the level of the distraught father (in this case the floor), the chaplain was able to encourage the father to face his own responsibility in the tragic case and start to build a new relationship with God. The father concludes 'It's my fault, I've killed Claire, the only one I've really loved. Why doesn't God take me?' (Speck, 1988). As Kreidler points out:

'An authentic man is responsible to himself and to a power greater than himself – God – however defined, for the choices he makes in life, the attitudes he forms, the use he makes of his potential and gifts, and the living in the "now" of each moment. Man cannot live authentically if he sees himself as powerless.'

(Kreidler, 1984)

Empowering those who see themselves as 'defeated' is one of the constructs of a healing presence. The apparently powerless patient or relative starts to heal only when they can begin to crystallise their emotions, challenge their gods and put their lives and concerns into a cosmic perspective, for it is the angered, frightened soul who screams accusingly, yet *resignedly* at God.

Humour

Yet another avenue of caring that is open to nurses who are confronted with patients in spiritual and psychological distress is humour. Humour as a subconstruct of caring is mentioned quite regularly, especially by nurses, as a manifestation of caring conduct. Humour is quite evident as a vehicle for commenting on the misfortune of those who are ill or in hospital, as witnessed by the variety of get well cards. Cards with humour can range from those consisting of cartoons with healthy good puns to quite raunchy, sexually abusive and stereotypical cards, which tend to be offensive and/or hurtful. Language too has a variety of humorous idioms that can be used in times of physical and psychological ailments and distress, and of course there is a vast array of jokes with more or less appropriate constructive humour.

Speck, however, additionally describes a form of patient, self-applied black humour (macabre, gallows humour) that can sometimes be effectively used in dispelling acute spiritual anxiety. A rather henpecked husband commented to him, in his role as hospital chaplain, that when he dies his wife will have him cremated and 'put in an hourglass. So I'll even have to work after I've gone!' (Speck, 1988). Likewise, patients with artificial limbs or prosthesis often joke about these appendages, but the attentive nurse should be capable of picking out when the humour is simply masking deep-seated sadness and/or revulsion.

The author has a relative who has an artifical limb, due to losing his arm during World War II attempting to blow up a tank in order to defend a column of resistance-fighters. This relative has often made macabre jokes of the gallows humour variety about his prosthesis to the author and yet to all intents and purposes leads a fulfilled and very active life with his one remaining arm and residual internal damage. Once, in recalling some wartime escapades, he shocked the author by calmly stating the equivalent of: 'Oh, I lost my arm at 9 o'clock on a Tuesday morning, the 19th September 1944'. The exact timing and date of this obviously significant event in his life was etched for ever in his memory, and his displays of humour were just another mechanism to help him come to terms with this enormous loss, in spite of apparently exceptionally good and effective adaptation to the situation.

A nurse would be well advised, therefore, not to assume too much or take too much for granted in regard to at least some forms of patient humour, especially of the self-depreciating variety. The mother who jokingly refers to her little toddler as her 'banana' due to the colour of its skin, caused by end stage biliary atresia, is fooling few people, although she may be humouring herself in a situation where she finds there is little else she can do. Again it is Speck, in commenting on the positive aspects of humour in pastoral care, who recalls the case of a dismayed mother-to-be, who had just found out that she was carrying triplets. She went to the Sister's office to attend Sunday Communion Service but because of her size decided to continue standing, propping up her large bulge on Sister's desk to relieve the weight. She was quite tearful. When the chaplain reached the words: '"Come unto me all ye who labour, and I will give you rest, there was a moment's silence and then both began to laugh and had great difficulty in regaining control'. As Speck comments, 'Far from being irreverent, the laughter transformed the situation and, after receiving the sacrament, the mother-to-be was noticeably calmer and more relaxed.' (Speck, 1988).

Certainly some chaplains and priests the author is acquainted with routinely finish their pastoral visits or healing sessions with a farewell parting joke, which has the property of concluding and efficiently closing a therapeutic session on a lighter note, yet without making the patient feel they are the butt of the humour. It is never at or about the patient that the nurse or health-care worker laughs, rather humour is used to defray tension and disperse some of the psychic energy and spiritual distress that is ever present. The nurse laughs with the patient, rather than because of the patient or at the patient's expense.

The author knows a gentleman with multiple sclerosis who is now in the final stages of the disease. He is wheel-chair bound and dependent on nursing staff for all his bodily needs and self-care activities. He is also prone to losing his voice which for him is doubly sad as he once had a strong lyrical voice and enjoyed singing in the choir. This disabled friend is in the habit of telephoning the author at home with the help of his POSSUM (from latin, 'I can') and once having made the telephone connection attempts to make a conversation.

The problem lies in the fact that very often all the author can hear is extremely heavy breathing and panting over the phone, usually followed by electronic whirls and buzzings, as he tries to raise his voice and/or amplify the few sounds which he can produce. One day, upon visiting him, I said, 'You do realise that you sound extremely lecherous over the phone, and God forbid I should get a real such annoyance call, for all the astonished person on the other end of the phone would hear would be my emphatic insistence that they "speak up, and take their time!"' My friend laughed heartily until he was quite red in the face and tears of mirth were in his eyes. Laughing at the absurdity of the situation made light of his distress and utter humiliation, where even talking over the phone was becoming a problem for him. Humour in such instances can say as much as many words and much non-verbal language. No need to acknowledge the level of spiritual distress here, where all that is left is the ability to laugh at the situation.

It hardly needs to be said that nurses using humour with patients need to be very careful as to how and with whom they apply it. The insistence of patients that nurses or visitors do not tell jokes because 'it hurts' is not exaggerated, and this also needs to be reckoned with. Finally the vulnerable, fragile patient experiencing acute distress may well find the potted humour of television if not distasteful, then certainly upon occasion hurtful, as this is not aimed at any special group of people but rather the average viewer, who is not considered to be ill, frail, infirm or in distress. It is therefore all the more ironic that televisions are often left switched on all day in busy wards – as the querulous guardians and keepers of distressed souls, causing untold harm and questionable good. As comments on the BBC's 'Does he take sugar' programme on Radio 4 can substantiate, humour in the mass media can be quite insulting and hurting towards disabled and ill patients.

Perhaps another form of caring would be for the more politically active nurses to complain to the appropriate authorities at inappropriate jokes, headline innuendos and cartoons. Certainly political activities have caring overtones and some forms of caring most definitely call for active political intervention. Humour can help in the healing process but when it is inappropriate it can also be damaging and very hurtful.

Nonetheless, as Cummings noted, 'who were so dark of heart they might not speak, a little innocence will make them sing' (Cummings, 1960). Similarly, Evely, commenting on the pathos of suffering adds that to recover from deep sadness and depression one needs to locate the focus of happiness, which often 'involves accepting to plunge again into our condition, out of which we are trying to escape' (Evely, 1967); or, as Sophocles philosophically observed in Antigone, 'life without life's joys is living death' (Sophocles, 1947).

Aamodt (1988), writing in Leininger's book on *Caring*, quotes a paralysed patient who says 'the pits of dependency is not being able to scratch yourself'. For such a patient the only joy left in this situation, as for my friend suffering with multiple-sclerosis, is to somehow find a way to laugh at the situation. Even the frail mentally ill may find it in themselves to laugh and see the humour of the situation, as the anonymous writer of the doggerel quoted by Cohen:

> 'My bifocals fit
> My dentures are fine
> My hearing aid works
> But I do miss my mind.'

(Cohen, 1990)

In conclusion, as Cohen noted in her fascinating article on the power of humour to heal and restore strength, 'it is essential to laugh with others, not at them . . . the need to laugh should be added to our basic needs for love, trust and security. To be healthy, mirth must occur within the context of understanding love and support' (Cohen, 1990).

Encouraging beauty

There is yet another way that the nurse can help the distressed mind and soul reach some equilibrium and thereby manifest caring, and this is by encouraging the presence of beauty. The human spirit and psyche is of its nature yearning for perfection and aesthetic beauty, and much has been written from the ancient Greeks to the present day on the nature of beauty and the quality of aestheticism. Suffice to say here that the human spirit would appear to react and function better in pleasing surroundings, in an aesthetically constructive milieu rather than in a drab monotonous environment bombarded with third rate stimulii that tend to depress and/or agitate the spirit rather than soothe and heal. The popular nursing literature is full of accounts of the effect of the environment on patients self-esteem and even increased rates of healing. Physiologists have long campaigned for hospital architects to construct patient areas with windows and vistas on nature, if not direct access to the outside world; for the human spirit together with the soma combines to function more effectively when it is more in synchrony with the natural time of day, seasons of the year, and has access to the beauties and wonders of nature.

There is much anecdotal evidence that the presence of beauty accompanies and accelerates the healing process and it may prove a fruitful area for future nursing research. Certainly it is more pleasant and conducive to caring if a patient is nursed in a beautiful setting, where the walls are aesthetically painted, the floors are clean, sounds are muffled and the seasons of the year mark their progress from outside large picture windows.

The author remembers well visits to a relative in an intensive care unit where from outside the huge bay windows the warm May sun had called forth the early spring flowers. In the distance the snow-capped mountains stood witness to the passing of spent lives, and the pet sheepdog of one of the patients, oblivious to the sonority of the view, sat on guard outside the window, occasionally frolicking around the field as if to reassert the painfully obvious truth that life must and will go on. There was something gentle and soothing about that intrusion of nature into the high technology of the unit and especially at night-time when the presence of the stars, like a thousand lights, reminded the staff and relatives of patients on that busy unit that they too had a part to play in the vast canvas of the ever-unfolding universe.

Leininger quotes just such sentiments by a resident poet at the Colorado Caring Sciences Unit who observed for a while the work of midwives. The poet wrote of those transcendental moments following birth, so similar in intensity to those often accompanying death, that even masters of words and emotions can note the confusion, as Eliot in the Three Magi wrote of the human spirit impinging on cosmic truths:

> ' . . . I had seen birth and death,
> But had thought they were different; this Birth was
> Hard and bitter agony for us, like Death; our death.'
>
> (Eliot, 1963)

It was considerably easier to feel at one with the universe in that environment, and to tap the energies of self-awareness, than in an intensive care unit also frequented by the author in a large cos-mopolitan city where the colour of the walls was not visible for the amount of equipment lining them; no windows were available to indicate the seasons, weather, or time of day, and the ultra-sanitised environment discouraged displays of normal human affection, such as holding the patient's hand or even covering them up with a warm blanket. Somehow the patient was lost in the hardware and medical paraphernalia. As one distraught mother said, looking at her child in an intensive care cot, 'I cannot touch him, this is not my child'. She did not recognise her child in all the equipment. She was lost and was rejecting the foreignness that confronted her.

Virginia Henderson, commenting on the apparent lack of basic caring skills by nurses in such environments, queries the education and health-care system that encourages such apparent callousness (Hen-derson, 1980). Perhaps it is not just a matter of inadequate preparation for the work to be done and the presence of a health-care system inconducive to manifestations of intra-human caring; perhaps the very lack of an atmosphere of beauty and aesthetically pleasing surround-ings has also a part to play. When the human psyche and spirit is suffering, the presence of beauty is especially important. How is one to convince a disillusioned depressed patient that they matter and are intrinsically important to us and to themselves when they are nursed in an environment that few of us would wish to live or stay in.

If the ancient Greeks saw fit to build their healing temples in the most beautiful locations in the Aegean Sea that they could find, perhaps we too could learn something from them about the significance of beauty in the healing process. Beauty however, should not be just confined to walls and external environment. Beauty as a manifestation and indeed reflection of caring should encompass such aspects as the patients' and staffs' personal dignity; e.g., wearing of appropriate and pleasing clothing, maintaining an odour-free environment, removing from sight needless reminders of dependency and stress, such as commodes and bedpans. All of this in total makes up a harmonious whole that strives to approximate normal home-like living and introduce an element of beauty around the patient that aims to elevate the spirit, rather than depress it or ignore its needs and concerns.

Even in the most drab of surroundings healing beauty can be consciously introduced, via bouquets of flowers and plants or giving a patient a beautiful or insightful book to read that can truly elevate the spirit as the effect of Moustakas' book on loneliness had on many of his patients and spiritually distraught people. Music can be introduced which can unite and be efficacious where words are quite meaningless. Caring for the spirit, however, by paying attention to the deliberate promotion of beauty is neither easy nor simple, but certainly worth some effort and time.

Empowering hope

The object of all these manifestations of caring that are aimed at helping the spirit and psyche to start to heal itself is to introduce into the total telic disintegration an element of hope. As Kreidler in her article on the *Meaning of Suffering* notes, for those especially suffering spiritual and psychic distress in addition to physical ailments 'meaning may be discovered when one learns how to love, trust, hope, forgive or be forgiven . . . for life is a task which requires a human response . . . yet man cannot live authentically if he sees himself as powerless' (Kreidler, 1984). Embuing patients with hope and empowering them to see meaning in suffering is the ultimate and most difficult task of the professional and practising holistic nurse. As Kreidler continues:

> 'crisis, hardship and pain can cause man to suffer spiritually if they are viewed as meaningless. Once they are placed in a context of meaning they cease to be suffering . . . the patient may need adequate pain relief, information, skilled nursing care, or someone who inspires hope, trust and love in a situation which can initially be viewed as hopeless.'

So often it is the patient's view of his situation as one of hopelessness that triggers off the cascade of events that leads to spiritual disintegration and distress. Kreidler sees nursing as 'encouraging in all persons a sense of dignity, worth and power. It is based on the hope that human integrity as well as faith in the meaning of life itself will be preserved'. This empowering hope must be transmitted successfully from the nurse or health-care worker to the patient, otherwise the patient with a spinal cord injury will see no point in physiotherapy, the new amputee will not contemplate re-integration into society and the youngster paralysed from the neck down, due to a road traffic accident, will see no logical need to attend school and study for exams. Life will hold no meaning for them as all of their life is seen to be focused on that which is humanly speaking indeed meaningless. What should be viewed as a whole will be reduced to that which is missing, defective or diseased.

According to Watson, to inspire hope in a patient is one of the central basic assumptions of the science of caring in nursing, and is one of her 10 carative factors that 'form a structure for studying and understanding nursing . . . ' (Watson, 1985). Watson sees the installation of faith-hope as pivotal to patient healing and a central caring phenomena for:

> 'installation of faith-hope in one's self and one's competence, or in another person, is incorporated into the science of caring. The healing power of belief should never be overlooked . . . the holistic nature of responding to another person justifies faith-hope as a contributing influence in people's lives.'
>
> (Watson, 1985)

Since nurses are encroaching, infringing and often directly manipulating people's lives, it seems appropriate that they also look at the properties of faith and hope and evaluate their roles in practice.

The philosopher Mayeroff in the early 1970s wrote a short monograph, *On Caring*, and this work of his helped launch the many nurse theoreticians' subsequent tracts on caring. In this work Mayeroff viewed hope as one of the major constructs of caring, together with knowledge, patience, honesty, trust, humility, courage and the ability to adapt or adjust. The hope that he referred to is the hope 'that the other will grow through my caring . . . it is akin, in some ways, to the hope that accompanies the coming of spring' (Mayeroff, 1971). He rightfully pointed out that this hope has nothing to do with wishful thinking and unfounded expectations, rather 'it is an expression of the plenitude of the present, a present alive with a sense of the possible'. Since Mayeroff sees inter and intra personal growth as the measure *and* criteria for caring, it is not surprising that he states 'where there is no possibility of new growth, there is despair'. The couple who lost both their children in tragic circumstances, despite the crushing agony that this must have represented to them, did not despair but rather hoped. They saw in each other *life* and energy; they saw potential for growth, and by caring for each other ultimately managed to integrate the losses into some meaningful structure in their lives, and even ultimately found the energy within themselves to reach out and offer hope and power to others. This healing hope, according to Mayeroff, 'rallies energies and activates our powers; it is not a passive waiting for something to happen from outside'. In fact my role in offering hope in this instance was minimal. The powers to heal were in them themselves.

The depressed, totally spiritually disorganised and decentralised individuals, are however totally bereft of hope. In such cases the nurse may find that she needs to literally share her own hope with the other, and this may be in the face of the patient's sullen anger and/or professional mistrust or incomprehension. It may demand of her much courage. As Mayeroff observes, 'despair militates against courage, it drains it of vitality'. It is not easy then to hope and to trust in one's vision when all one's colleagues are dubious and prone to ridicule one, and the patient is totally passive. This point is eloquently brought out in Kipling's immortal poem, 'If'. As Mayeroff elaborates, 'it is not simply hope for the other, it is hope for the realisation of the other through my caring . . . ' This indeed may take courage, and:

'such courage is found in standing by the other in trying circumstances, and in taking risks that go beyond safety and security, (for) if I did not believe that I would stand up for the other in difficult circumstances, my hope for the growth of the other through my caring would be necessarily undermined.'

The patient *must* be convinced that I care enough about him to, in the phrase of Hutchinson, be prepared to engage in 'responsible subversion' should that be necessary (Hutchinson, 1990). I should be prepared to do that, because I have trust in my patients and I see hope for them and within them. Rawnsley, in an article looking at the ethics of meaningful nursing research comments that nursing is:

'an opportunity to know joy and sadness, love and desire and even pain, and the courage to face that pain. Perhaps life's greatest promise is the hope of transcending self-absorption and really experiencing each other.'

(Rawnsley, 1985)

Hope helps the distressed patient to transcend self-absorption by not only looking beyond themselves but also by offering a basis for the courage to look within themselves.

Pepper, in a centennial address to cancer nurses, and published in *Cancer Nursing*, analyses the ingredients which he saw present in the caring behaviours of a group of nurses who worked with survivors of cancer and described in his book, *We the Victors* (Pepper, 1985). He saw caring, love, and hope, as the three active ingredients that made qualitative differences to the lives of these 'survivors'. He comments that it was as if 'they were caring for something more than the lives of their patients, something I call life within life itself'. Nurses offered empowering hope to their devastated cancer patients and watched what he refers to as the 'trinity of care and love and hope' take fruition. Interestingly, he thought that the nurses offered firstly care, then love, and lastly hope, in a sequential order, as if it was the existence of caring behaviours that empowered love to be shared that ultimately allowed hope the room to blossom.

Hall, in a recent article looking at the effect of hope on the diagnosed terminally ill person found that her informants, in spite of periodic and to be expected set-backs, all regained a measure of hope in the face of a certain diagnosis of terminal illness, and this was achieved not by information-seeking, which could have been a form of external justification for unrealistic wishful thinking, but by affect-control strategies, that were self-originating and empowering processes (Hall, 1990). She quotes them as referring to their (often) new-found hope, as having 'transformed the shame into pride about the things that I can accomplish, and the effectiveness of my state of mind has helped some other that I know . . . ' or 'part of my attitude is that we are all going to be alive only as long as we are going to be alive and there is not a thing we can do to change that fact?' or 'don't feel like a victim. You can live with it' (Hall, 1990). These patients are all expressing the empowerment that the presence of hope can bring to bear on an otherwise 'hopeless' situation. These patients, Hall states, in accordance with other studies, defined hope as having a future life in spite of the diagnosis, having a renewed zest for life, finding a reason for living that often was not present before, and *trusting* the health-care provider to stand beside them. Such a definition of hope has universal application in the health-care system and it is these properties of hope and trust that the nurse is asked, by Watson and others, to instil creatively in those patients who are without hope. All too often however, as Hall observed, 'hope is deemed a form of denial or false reality, instead of a universal need of humans . . . ' Without the presence of hope, the spiritually and psychologically distressed patients will not find the energy to start creatively to grow and re-orientate themselves.

Prayer

It would be odd, if in a chapter on the caring aspects of spiritual and psychological distress some space was not given to the healing effects of prayer. Prayer from time immemorial and in all religions and cultures has always played a large role in the amelioration of suffering and distress, especially spiritual and psychological distress (Dugan, 1987/88; McGlone, 1990; Taylor and Ferszt, 1990; Leggieri, 1986). The official presence of hospital chaplains in our major medical centres attests to the fact that we acknowledge the existence of the spirit and the importance for some patients and staff of spiritual and psycho-cultural matters (Leggieri, 1986; Speck, 1988; Campbell, 1985; Campbell, 1984). Interest in the healing of the spirit has increased recently among nurses, encouraged no doubt by the holistic nature of the caring theories that include care of the spirit among their primary objectives (Watson, 1985; Rogers, 1980; Beeny, 1990). Caring for the spirit has been the subject of this chapter, and it now is imperative, however briefly, to examine some ideas about the role that prayer may have in healing the wounded spirit, and how the nurse might employ prayer, in helping the spirit to heal.

Prayer is a profoundly personal act, a point of personal union between mortal man and a Transcendent Spirit. Various religions have prescribed how that moment of union may take place, often combining elements of vocal supplication with prescribed gestures and even in some instances suggesting times of day that these states of union are to take place.

In Western Christian-Judaic tradition the Transcendent Spirit is seen as an omnipotent, omnipresent and above all compassionate, personal God, and therefore prayer is seen as an effort in reaching out to God, and in establishing contact. According to Merton, prayer can be seen as:

'a deep personal integration in an attentive, watchful listening of "the heart". The response such prayer calls forth is not usually one of jubilation or audible witness; it is a wordless and total surrender of the heart in silence.'

(Merton, 1971)

Although the Christian-Judaic tradition, like other great religious traditions puts a strong emphasis on communal verbal prayer, as evidenced by various paraliturgical services, group recitations of prescribed prayers, litanies and, in the Roman Catholic tradition, group recitation of the rosary, by far an even greater emphasis is put on the cultivation of quiet prayer, especially in relation to healing the spirit. The vast body of literature on mystical prayer and the central role that quiet prayer is seen to play in the life of an individual attests to the fact that what really counts in spiritual wellbeing is not the amount of words used in prayer or the volume of the words, but the quality of contact established between the spirit and a transcendent God. The insistence on the value of quiet prayer has significant implications for healing the broken spirit. Whereas praying aloud with a person is a form of acknowledging spiritual distress, and often healing sessions in a religious context, such as within the charismatic movement, are accompanied by obvious verbal prayers, no real healing can take place unless the person suffering or someone on their behalf establishes contact with God, that is the individual personally experiences the reality of prayer.

The primary object of this type of prayer is to prepare the individual to see himself as he really is, a form of religious introspection, that in the Christian tradition culminates in the awareness that we are all in need of forgiveness and need to forgive; initially ourselves, and then others. When this point of awareness is reached, prayer becomes an open dialogue with God, or some form of Transcendency. Until the person in spiritual distress reaches this awareness, it is difficult for him to be open to the healing powers of prayer.

As Dom Heron in his book on spiritual healing and the efficacy of prayer on physical and psychological healing states:

> 'I normally start by praying for spiritual and mental or emotional healing before I pray for the well-being of the body. This seems to be the right way round, not only because spiritual healing is the most important area of healing, but also because spiritual and mental or emotional sickness quite often cause physical sickness, and quite often the physical healing will not take place until people have been healed at the other levels.'
>
> (Heron, 1989)

If prayer is seen as such a personal event, how can a nurse confronted with the patient in spiritual and psychological distress attempt to intervene with prayer? Firstly, as with all attention surrounding spiritual and psychological disintegration, the nurses' awareness of the benefit of prayer and its importance for the patient is in itself therapeutic. Thus, because the nurse knows and is aware of the benefits of prayer, she will give the patient time and space to foster his own prayer life, even within the confines of a busy acute-care hospital ward. Allowing a patient to finish reading his prayers, to allow another to set up a prayer mat and pray quietly in the corner of the ward, to put on purposefully a Sunday worship programme on TV for those patients who request it; all these actions contribute to acknowledging that prayer and an active prayer life all have a role to play in healing the spirit.

For the hurting, frightened patient, prayer helps focus the distressed floundering Spirit. Patients also may ask the nurse to pray with them or arrange for the procurement of some item of piety. Praying with a patient, however, will only be possible if the nurse herself is comfortable with her own spirituality and has a repetoire of applicable prayers that she feels at ease in sharing. The prayers should be recognisable to the patient and reflect the patient's own spirituality, for there is little room in healing the spirit for insincerity and 'pious dishonesty'. Prayer unites people at a level that physical presence rarely can accomplish. Since the healing presence of prayer is to some extent separate from the intrinsic worth of those who pray, the nurse, providing she is sincere in her intentions, cannot transgress 'spiritual norms'. Providing the prayer is meaningful and not solely a rote duty in fulfilment of patients' wishes, then its efficacy can be assured. As Tennyson observed, 'more things are wrought by prayer than this world dreams of . . . ' (Tennyson, 1983).

The nurse, however, may feel she indeed cannot 'pray' with a patient but that she can only be quietly present while a patient prays, if he so wishes. In the final eventuality she can suggest someone else to pray with the patient, whom she feels is more qualified to pray than herself, but automatically calling for 'the padre' or the vicar should not be encouraged (Speck, 1988; Leggieri, 1986; McGlone, 1990). Everyone has a spirit with their own unique prayerlife. Prayer is for the spirit what food is for the some. The spirit needs prayer for its wellbeing and nourishment. As a sixteenth century Spanish mystic observed:

> 'Souls without prayer are like people whose bodies or limbs are paralysed; they possess feet and hands but they cannot control them.'
>
> (Teresa of Avila, 1961).

It is not, as mentioned previously, quantity or even objective value of words that will constitute the nature of prayer; rather, the amount of self put into the attempt at reaching the Spirit and the Transcendency that the Spirit represents, is what will determine the nature of the prayerful encounter of the soul with its creator. Although many nurses may initially feel uncomfortable when praying with patients, because nourishing and mending broken spirits via prayer is the work of all individuals, (however unconsciously) towards self-caring of the spirit; the experience should not have to jar too abruptly for too long. Indeed as C. S. Lewis notes:

> ' . . . all prayers blaspheme worshipping with frail images a folklore dream, and all men in their praying, self-deceived, address the coinage of their own unquiet thoughts . . . '
>
> (Etchells, 1990)

Nonetheless, the power of prayer for the spiritually distressed is undeniable. Evidence in the nursing and health-care literature suggests that once nurses are asked to participate in the prayer life and spiritual domain of their patients, they tend not to regret the experience (Speck, 1987; Campbell, 1985; McFarlane, 1988; Heron, 1989). Ultimately, if prayer and praying is important and central to the lives of our patients, it should be important and significant to health-care providers also, 'for what are men better than sheep or goats that nourish a blind life within the brain, if knowing God, they lift not hands of prayer . . . ' (Tennyson, 1983).

Prayer life can be sustained and encouraged by various para-liturgical ceremonies, devotionals, sacramentals, and by the administration of sacraments. In the Judaeo-Christian tradition (and in several other religions) the sick are particularly cared for due to the long tradition of caring for the sick and wounded. Currently, for Christians within the sacrament of the sick there are established liturgical healing rites for the sick and ailing. For Christians the sacrament of the sick, administered by a hospital chaplain who is actively engaged in the business of healing wounded spirits and frightened ailing bodies, has the power not only in its inherent sacramental value (for a long time seen as appropriate to instil peace of mind and soul for those considered to be dying), but it also has unique healing properties in its own right and hence very appropriate for those considered in need of spiritual and psychological healing (Heron, 1989; Taylor and Ferszt, 1990).

The sacrament of the sick, administered together with a healing rite, can have enormous benefits to all those who are sick or are considered potentially ill such as patients prior to surgery, and those with chronic diseases (Heron, 1989). The presence of a nurse during the administration of the sacrament of the sick, and her presence during a healing ceremony, can have positive effects on patients and is often perceived as a humbling yet exhilarating experience by health-care workers (Heron, 1989; McGlone, 1990; Taylor and Ferszt, 1990). Few actions unite health-care workers and patients together so effectively as prayer and praying for spiritual and psychological healing, since faced with transcendental Truths any perceived apparent differences between the cared-for and caring disappear (Kreidler, 1984; Oliver, 1990).

As Mayeroff and others have observed, growth can only start taking place in the caring act when both the cared for and the carer perceive the need for each other, for improvement and for progress (Mayeroff, 1971). Restoration of spiritual well-being, often via prayer and healing services, is as much a need of the patient as it is of the health-care workers. Restoration of spiritual equilibrium is a mutually necessary condition for total well-being; a goal of all holistic nursing practice theories. As Speck notes in his monograph, (1988) patients are often surprised and touched when they find out that 'others' are praying for them and often observe 'But I'm not a practising Christian' or 'I'm not a Christian at all'. Nonetheless, the majority of patients of whatever religion or spiritual inclination do seem to appreciate the degree of love and attention that praying for and with someone implies.

Interestingly, patients and clients of non-Christian traditions appreciate when attention is paid to their spiritual needs; and, although it may be hard or impossible for a Christian nurse to pray with an Islamic patient, providing the space for them to pray and being a silent but spiritually active witness when they pray can also help create the healing, unitive climate of spiritual integration and manifestation of human concern. The author recalls that some of her most memorable nursing moments were when she was praying with patients, during times of birth or death or other personal crises of the patients. One of her most spiritually meaningful periods was when she prayed with Islamic children on an oncology unit. Here, in the absence of a common language, culture, tradition, educational background or even religion, what bound the children to the nurse and the nurse to the children were the quiet moments spent in prayer. The children knew I was not a Muslim, but I prayed in silence beside them, while they chanted in harmony, and as a group we were secure in the knowledge that we were united in purpose and goal. Such moments of true prayer are not forgotten easily, for to touch the Godhead in prayer is a rare and precious occasion, and in all religious traditions the innocent prayer of children has a special powerful significance.

In conclusion, while addressing aspects of spiritual distress present among patients, it is important not to forget the curative role of prayer in the healing process, and it is important also to foster an approach to personal spirituality which provides meaning to the nurses' life (Steeves and Kahn, 1987; Burnard, 1990; Kreidler, 1984; McFarlane, 1988). In the course of working through one's life's meaning and establishing a personal and professional philosophy, quiet moments of reflection or prayer have an important role to fulfil. Rather than avoid eschatological questions and skirt transcendental issues of life and death, the nurse should repeatedly go back to them, learning from practice and experience how to integrate eventful, pivotal moments into meaningful life-bearing powers and energy. Certainly in many of the major world religions this self-actualising and growing process is facilitated by fostering a personal prayer life and/or respect for reflexive transcendental moments of others.

Conclusion

Contemporary thinking in nursing care challenges the practising professional to re-examine his or her beliefs, attitudes and knowledge base, for ethical viability and clinical credibility. The growing awareness that nursing professionals, as indeed all members of the helping professions, will need to continuously update their practice based on current research and professional debate, is not difficult to understand or justify.

The philosophies held by nurses, their awareness of the political and social context within which they deliver care and their familiarity with the attitudes towards nursing theory, models of nursing, and the nursing process will all influence the quality of the care they deliver. Augmented with the efficient use of modern technologies, artificial intelligence, and information technologies, this care should reflect excellence of practice. Nursing sciences in such a framework will reflect a considerate, reflective, and sensitive approach to patient and client care, which is the only ultimate rationale for professional intervention.

This approach calls for a challenge to change from nursing based on yesterday's norms to nursing with a view to future, anticipated needs. For caring to be truly present it should be characterised by its pro-active stance. It is the anticipated and expected needs of the patient that should be addressed most urgently now, rather than heroic activities enacted once the patient is thoroughly incapacitated. This is contemporary thinking in nursing care – the new challenge to change.

References

Aamodt, A. M. (1988). Themes and issues in conceptualizing care. In: *Care: the Essence Of Nursing and Health*. M. M. Leininger (Ed), pp. 75–9. Wayne State University Press, Detroit.

Bakan, D. (1968). *Disease, Pain and Sacrifice: Towards a Psychology Of Suffering*. Beacon Press, Boston.

Bambrough, R. (Ed), (1963). *The Philosophy of Aristotle*. New American Library, New York.

Beeny, J. (1990). Primary Health Care. Spiritual healing. *Nursing Standard*, **5(11)**, 48–9.

Benner, P. (1984). *From Novice to Expert*. Addison-Wesley, Menlo Park.

Bergman, R. (1983). Understanding the patient in all his human needs. *Journal of Advanced Nursing*, **8(3)**, 185–90.

Burnard, P. (1987). Spiritual distress and the nursing response: theoretical considerations and counselling skills. *Journal of Advanced Nursing*, **12(3)**, 377–82.

Burnard, P. (1990). Learning to care for the spirit. *Nursing Standard*, **4(18)**, 38–9.

Campbell, A. V. (1984). *Moderated Love*. SPCK, London.

Campbell, A. V. (1985). *Paid to Care? The Limits Of Professionalism in Pastoral Care*. SPCK, London.

Campbell, A. V. (1988). Profession and vocation. In: *Ethical Issues in Caring*. G. Fairbairn and S. Fairbairn (Eds), pp. 1–9. Avebury, Aldershot.

Cohen, M. (1990). Caring for ourselves can be funny business. *Holistic Nursing Practice*, **4(4)**, 1–11.

Cummings, E. E. (1960). *Selected Poems 1923–1958*. Faber and Faber, London.

Dugan, D. O. (1987/88). Essays on the art of caring in nursing 1. The human spirit in stress management. *Nursing Forum*, **23(3)**, 108–17.

Eliot, T. S. (1963). *Collected Poems 1909–1962*. Faber and Faber, London.

Etchells, R. (Comp) (1990). *Praying With the English Poets*. SPCK, London.

Evely, L. (1967). *Suffering*. Herder and Herder, New York.

Gaylin, W. (1985). Feelings. In: *Powers That Make Us Human: the Foundations Of Medical Ethics*. K. Vaux (Ed), pp. 55–73. University of Illinois Press, Chicago.

Habel, N. C. (Ed), (1975). *Book of Job*. Cambridge University Press, London. (The Cambridge Bible Commentary).

Hall, B. A. (1990). The struggle of the diagnosed terminally ill person to maintain hope. *Nursing Science Quarterly*, **3(4)**, 177–84.

Henderson, V. (1978). The concept of nursing. *Journal of Advanced Nursing*, **3(2)**, 113–30.

Henderson, V. (1980). Preserving the essence of nursing in a technological age. *Journal of Advanced Nursing*, **5(3)**, 245–60.

Heron, B. (1989). *Praying For Healing: the Challenge*. Darton, Longman and Todd, London.

Hopkins, G. M. (1953). *Selected Poems*. Heinemann, London.

Hutchinson, S. A. (1990). Responsible subversion: a study of rule bending among nurses. *Scholarly Inquiry for Nursing Practice*, **4(1)**, 3–17.

Kreidler, M. (1984). Meaning in suffering. *International Nursing Review*. **31(6)**, 174–6.

Laburn, E. (1988). Spiritual care: an element in nursing care planning. *Journal of Advanced Nursing*, **13(3)**, 314–20.

Leggieri, J. (1986). Pastoral care in the hospital: uniqueness and contribution. *Topics in Clinical Nursing*, **8(2)**, 47–55.

Leininger, M. M. (1981). The phenomenon of caring: importance, research questions and theoretical considerations. In: *Caring: An Essential Human Need. Proceedings of Three National Caring Conferences*. M. M. Leininger, (Ed), pp. 3–14. Slack, Thorofare.

Liehr, P. R. (1989). The core of true presence: a loving center. *Nursing Science Quarterly*, **2(1)**, 7–8.

Martin, B. (1959). *No one must ever know*. Garden City, Doubleday Co.

May, R. (1977). *The meaning of anxiety*. Rev. edn. Norton, New York.

Mayeroff, M. (1971). *On Caring*. Harper and Row, New York.

McFarlane, J. (1988). Nursing: a paradigm of caring. In: *Ethical Issues In Caring*. G. Fairbairn and S. Fairbairn (Eds), pp. 10–20. Avebury, Aldershot.

McGlone, M. E. (1990). Healing the spirit. *Holistic Nursing Practice*, **4(4)**, 77–84.

Merton, T. (1971). *Contemplative Prayer*. Doubleday, New York.

Montagu, A. (1971). *Touching*. Harper and Row, New York.

Moustakas, C. (1975). *The Touch Of Loneliness*. Prenctice-Hall, Englewood Cliffs.

Oliver, N. R. (1990). Nurse, are you a healer? *Nursing Forum*, **25(2)**, 11–4.

Parse, R. R. (1981). Caring from a human science perspective. In: *Caring: An Essential Human Need. Proceedings of Three National Caring Conferences*. M. M. Leininger (Ed), pp. 129–32. Slack, Thorofare.

Parse, R. R. (1989). Essentials for practising the art of nursing. *Nursing Science Quarterly*, **2(3)**, 111.

Pepper, C. B. (1985). The roles of care and love and hope between nurse and patient in cancer survival. *Cancer Nursing,* **8**(Suppl. 1), 50–3.

Pratt, J. W. and Mason, A. (1981). *The Caring Touch*. HM & M, London.

Rawnsley, M. M. (1985). Nursing: the compassionate science. *Cancer Nursing*, 8, Supplement 1, 71–4.

Robbins, C. (1991). Body, mind and spirit. *Nursing: the Journal of Clinical Practice, Education and Management*, **4(31)**, 9–11.

Rogers, M. E. (1980). Nursing: a science of unitary man. In: *Conceptual Models For Nursing*, 2nd edn. J. Riehl and C. Roy (Eds), pp. 329–37. Appleton-Century-Crofts, New York.

Saint-Exupery, A. de (1974). *The Little Prince*. Pan, London.

St Vincent Millay, E. (1964). *Collected Lyrics*. Washington Square Press, New York.

Sophocles, (1947). *The Theban Plays*, Penguin, Harmondsworth.

Speck, P. (1988). *Being There: Pastoral Care In Time Of Illness*. SPCK, London.

Steeves, R. H. and Kahn, D. L. (1987). Experience of meaning in suffering. *Image*, **19(3)**, 114–6.

Stoll, R. I. (1979). Guidelines for spiritual assessment. *American Journal of Nursing*, **79(9)**, 1574–7.

Taylor, P. B. and Ferszt, G. G. (1990). Spiritual healing. *Holistic Nursing Practice*, **4(4)**, 32–8.

Tennyson, A. (1983). *Idylls Of the King*. Penguin, Harmondsworth.

Teresa of Avila. (1961). *Interior Castle*. Translated by E. A. Peers, Doubleday, New York.

Watson, J. (1985). *Nursing: the Philosophy and Science Of Caring*. Little, Brown, Boston.

Watson, M. J. (1988). New dimensions of human caring theory. *Nursing Science Quarterly*, **1(4)**, 175–81.

Index

263